Supervision in Social Work

Supervision is currently a "hot topic" in social work. The editors of this volume, both social work educators and researchers, believe that good supervision is fundamental to the development and maintenance of effective practice in social work. Supervision is seen as a key vehicle for continuing development of professional skills, the safeguarding of competent and ethical practice and oversight of the wellbeing of the practitioner. As a consequence the demand for trained and competent supervisors has increased and a perceived gap in availability can create a call for innovation and development in supervision. This book offers a collection of chapters which contribute new insights to the field. Authors from Australia and New Zealand, where supervision inquiry is strong, offer research-informed ideas and critical commentary with a dual focus on supervision of practitioners and students. Topics include external and interprofessional supervision, retention of practitioners, practitioner resilience and innovation in student supervision. This book will be of interest to supervisors of both practitioners and students and highly relevant to social work academics.

This book was originally published as a special issue of *Australian Social Work*.

Liz Beddoe is an Associate Professor in Social Work at the University of Auckland, New Zealand. Her teaching and research interests include critical perspectives on social work education, professional supervision, the professionalization of social work, interprofessional learning and various workforce issues.

Jane Maidment is an Associate Professor in Social Work at the University of Canterbury, New Zealand. She researched the experience of student supervision for both her PhD and in a second investigation regarding how difference and diversity were addressed by supervisors and supervisees. The findings of these projects have been published in international journals. Jane has also provided supervision workshop input for social work practitioners and field educators extensively throughout Australia and within New Zealand.

Supervision in Social Work

Contemporary Issues

Edited by
Liz Beddoe and Jane Maidment

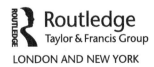

Routledge
Taylor & Francis Group

LONDON AND NEW YORK

First published 2015 by Routledge

2 Park Square, Milton Park, Abingdon, Oxon OX14 4RN
711 Third Avenue, New York, NY 10017, USA

Routledge is an imprint of the Taylor & Francis Group, an informa business

First issued in paperback 2017

British Library Cataloguing in Publication Data
A catalogue record for this book is available from the British Library

ISBN 13: 978-1-138-79923-3 (hbk)
ISBN 13: 978-1-138-05877-4 (pbk)

Typeset in Minion
by RefineCatch Limited, Bungay, Suffolk

Publisher's Note
The publisher accepts responsibility for any inconsistencies that may have
arisen during the conversion of this book from journal articles to book chapters,
namely the possible inclusion of journal terminology.

Disclaimer
Every effort has been made to contact copyright holders for their permission to
reprint material in this book. The publishers would be grateful to hear from any
copyright holder who is not here acknowledged and will undertake to rectify
any errors or omissions in future editions of this book.

Contents

Citation Information

The following chapters were originally published in *Australian Social Work*, volume 65, issue 2 (June 2012). When citing this material, please use the original page numbering for each article, as follows:

Chapter 2
Supervision is Not Politically Innocent
Carole Adamson
Australian Social Work, volume 65, issue 2 (June 2012) pp. 185–196

Chapter 3
External Supervision in Social Work: Power, Space, Risk, and the Search for Safety
Liz Beddoe
Australian Social Work, volume 65, issue 2 (June 2012) pp. 197–213

Chapter 4
Professional Supervision: A Workforce Retention Strategy for Social Work?
Phoebe Chiller & Beth R. Crisp
Australian Social Work, volume 65, issue 2 (June 2012) pp. 232–242

Chapter 5
Australian Social Work Supervision Practice in 2007
Ronnie Egan
Australian Social Work, volume 65, issue 2 (June 2012) pp. 171–184

Chapter 6
Windows on the Supervisee Experience: An Exploration of Supervisees' Supervision Histories
Kieran O'Donoghue
Australian Social Work, volume 65, issue 2 (June 2012) pp. 214–231

Chapter 9
Student Satisfaction with Models of Field Placement Supervision
Helen Cleak & Debra Smith
Australian Social Work, volume 65, issue 2 (June 2012) pp. 243–258

Please direct any queries you may have about the citations to
clsuk.permissions@cengage.com

Notes on Contributors

Carole Adamson is a Senior Lecturer in Social Work at the University of Auckland, New Zealand, where she teaches in social work and professional supervision programmes. A mental health practitioner, her main interests are in workplace stress, trauma, critical incidents, disaster and resilience, and how these knowledge bases can be embedded within the social work curriculum.

Liz Beddoe is an Associate Professor of Social Work at the University of Auckland, New Zealand. Her teaching and research interests include critical perspectives on social work education, professional supervision, and the media framing of social problems. She has published articles on supervision and professional issues in New Zealand and international journals.

Phoebe Chiller was completing a Bachelor of Social Work (Honours) degree in the School of Health and Social Development at Deakin University, Australia, at the time the research was conducted. She is now employed as a social worker at Barwon Youth in Geelong, Australia.

Helen Cleak is a Senior Lecturer in the Department of Social Work and Social Policy at La Trobe University, Australia. She teaches in social work practice skills and was the Director of Field Education and International Placements for over 20 years. Her book, co-authored with Jill Wilson, *Making the Most of Field Placement* is now in its 3rd edition and has been adopted as the major fieldwork text in most Australian social work courses.

Beth R. Crisp is a Professor in the School of Health and Social Development at Deakin University, Australia, where she is discipline leader for social work. Her research interests include areas of professional development and the transfer of professional knowledge.

Ronnie Egan is an Associate Professor of Field Education in the School of Global Urban and Social Studies at RMIT University, Melbourne, Australia. She has a practice history in the community sector including community health, sexual assault, and child and family relationships. Her research interests are in the areas of education, supervision and social work practice and teaching.

Jane Maidment is an Associate Professor in the Department of Human Services and Social Work at the University of Canterbury, New Zealand. She has had long standing involvement in field education research and co-ordination.

NOTES ON CONTRIBUTORS

Kieran O'Donoghue is an Associate Professor and Head of the School of Social Work at Massey University, New Zealand. He is a registered social worker and his main area of research is social work supervision.

Debra Smith is a Lecturer in Social Work in the School of Social Sciences at the University of Tasmania, Australia. She has a passion for social justice and is very active in the community. In recent years, her research interests have focused on social work education, in particular field education.

Acknowledgements

The editors would like to thank all the authors in this collection and to acknowledge the contribution made by Chris Bigby, as journal editor, to the special section on supervision which appeared in *Australian Social Work*, volume 65, issue 2.

Current Challenges in Supervision in Social Work

Liz Beddoe[a] & Jane Maidment[b]

[a]School of Counselling, Human Services and Social Work, University of Auckland, Auckland, New Zealand
[b]School of Language, Social and Political Sciences, University of Canterbury, Christchurch, New Zealand

Abstract

In 2012 Australian Social Work published a collection of articles focussed on current research and commentary on Australasian social work supervision, edited by Jane Maidment, Liz Beddoe and under the guiding eye of the journal's editor Christine Bigby (65(2)). It was the intention of the special section that the contents would "confirm the centrality of positive, learning focussed supervision, while fostering appropriate accountability and best practice in our discipline" (Maidment & Beddoe, 2012). Supervision has long been at the heart of professional development in social work and is a career-long commitment in our profession. Supervision provides a venue for diverse learning activities; a place and space where practitioners can refine their knowledge; develop skills and examine the challenges that are found in everyday practice. This chapter introduces the book and explores some recent developments in the scholarship and research of supervision.

Supervision is the main conduit for critically reflective practice but it is not the only vehicle for such development and it is important that we don't reify it. It is important therefore that we do not accept it uncritically and in our commentary introducing the special issue in 2012 we argued that it was necessary to interrogate current approaches and to continue to foster research and development. The six articles and the commentary in the special section were well received and have attracted a total of 5980 views (Taylor & Francis website) at the time of writing, we are pleased to note that they have attracted 70 citations (Google Scholar) and we are delighted that they are re-printed here in this collection. Our introductory chapter presents the contributions and introduces two new contributions.

In Chapter Seven in "Social Work Supervision for Changing Contexts", Liz Beddoe explores the significance of increasing requirements in supervision to be provided by trained and competent supervisors. A perception that there are too few well-prepared supervisors can create a call for more diversity in the modes of delivery of supervision, e.g., interprofessional, peer or group arrangements, as well as the "out-sourcing" to private practitioners. Such modes of supervision carry their own unique challenges and may also meet different needs at different stages of social worker careers. Drawing on the international literature and the author's own research the advantages and limitations of diverse approaches to supervision are explored.

In Chapter Eight, Jane Maidment provides guidance to field educators and students about how to develop their own practice framework during field placement supervision. In the chapter "Using Visual Cues to Develop a Practice Framework in Student Supervision" creating opportunities to use visual supports for learning in supervision are discussed. The notion of a practice framework is described followed by a discussion about how metaphor can enhance the learning associated with generating the framework. Student and field educator narratives about their experiences of developing a practice framework are included to illustrate.

Supervision: Organisational and Professional Dimensions

Supervision is a core practice activity in the social work profession and as such needs scholarly attention and research in order to build on current knowledge and extend it. In the commentary to the special section we argued that there was a need to "expand conceptual thinking about supervision; encourage innovation, and to capture new research in this field" (Maidment & Beddoe, 2012, p. 163). Six papers from the special issue are contained in this current volume, offering research and conceptual articles which provide original insights and critical perspectives on social work supervision. The contribution of these papers, and the further developments that have been reported in the intervening years, instils confidence that supervision research and development is thriving in Australia and New Zealand and is increasingly research-informed and reflective. Since 2012 further work has been published reporting evidence of a strong supervision research agenda present in Australia and New Zealand. The themes explored in this volume include critical, analytical perspectives on the state of supervision; the influence of practitioner experiences of supervision on supervisor practice; commentary on the politics of supervision and its focus within complex organisational environments; and the challenge to sustainability posed by traditional models of supervision in practice and field education.

We noted in 2012 that the scholarship of supervision was in good heart, evidenced by the number of books published on supervision and professional learning in social work, health and human services. Over the last two years many further publications have promoted supervision as a reflective space in which social work can be claimed and supported. In an era of austerity in social and health services there is some enthusiasm to move beyond a supervision discourse grounded in surveillance and risk management. Supervision has a role to play in all of the spheres in which social workers provide services.

There is a call for social work to stay faithful to its origins in addressing issues of social justice and oppression in the micro, mezzo and macro spheres. Baines, Charlesworth, Turner and O'Neill (2014, p. 6) note that some critical management literature discusses the potential that supervisors in social services can play an important role in "mediating impacts of managerialism on front-line staff and service users by using their organisational and discretionary power to challenge and destabilise the overarching dominance" of managerial practices. This approach explicitly positions supervisors in an organisational buffer zone, building on the mediative aspect of supervision first identified by Richards and Payne (1991) and later articulated by Morrison (2001) as engagement of supervisor and supervisee in exploring the complex and competing personal, organisational and professional agendas. Baines et al. (2014, p. 16) undertook comparative, international intensive case studies of changing work relations and the experience of front-line workers in the non-profit sector in Canada, Australia, Scotland and New Zealand and found that "strong supervision and an agency mission that is replete with social justice values" where managers are aligned with workers and community stakeholders can "buffer the demoralising aspects of lean care work".

The significance of supervision within our profession is highlighted by findings from two major national studies, one from Australia (Egan, 2012) and the other from New Zealand (O'Donoghue, 2012), both drawing on their doctoral research. Egan presents findings from a mixed methods quantitative study of supervision in Australia in 2007. Egan (2012, p.178) reports that 14.9% (86/579) of her respondents received external supervision and for 67.4% (391/580) their principal supervisor was also their line manager. Egan argues that organisational policy on supervision "requires an acknowledgement of these dual roles and the impact they have on accountability, conflicts of interest, confidentiality, contracts, performance appraisals, and finding the balance between the different functions of supervision" (2012, p. 180). She calls for further research to examine the organisational conditions where such dual roles occur to assess how compatible these arrangements are for effective supervision.

We note here also the contribution of Heather Hair's work in Canada, also reporting from a doctoral study (Hair, 2013; 2014 a; 2014b). Hair (2013, p. 1563) argues that in spite of the many claims made for supervision as essential for social work practice, four important issues have "been investigated and written about repeatedly, but without resolution". These issues concern the purpose of supervision, its duration over a career and aspects of the training and regulation of supervisors. Hair argues that it is vital that these often contested elements are developed to avoid erosion of supervision.

Supervision is currently recognised as being in a somewhat ambiguous position, on the one hand growing in importance; however this growth is not uncontested in its uneasy relationship with managerial concerns and organisational surveillance (Beddoe, 2010). In arguing that supervision might be situated as a "trade-off" between managerial and professional concerns Jones (2004, p. 12) argues that new public management has disrupted the stability of supervision while Noble and Irwin (2009) suggest that supervision has not been protected from the impact of the decades of restructuring in social work. The emphasis on managerial targets has the potential to reduce the impact of supervision as a professional space for reflection. In this collection Adamson (2012) asserts that supervision is not "politically innocent" and may be harnessed to compliance at the expense of the more clinically focused reflective supervision promoted in the literature. Adamson develops the metaphor of a "swingometer" to illustrate a supervision pendulum, which swings between a focus on social worker development and reflection and accountability driven "risk management". This is an international issue and in a three-country study Bradley, Engelbrecht and Höjer (2010) noted the predominance of administratively dominated supervision within management-driven social work agencies.

The growth of external supervision noted by many (see for example, Bradley et al., 2010; Bradley & Höjer, 2009), is in part motivated by unease with the power dynamics and bureaucratic nature of internal supervision provided by line managers, but often linked to the lack of suitably trained supervisors (Beddoe, 2010). External supervision may not be a panacea and should not escape critical interrogation and Beddoe (2011a) draws on Bernstein's notions of "vertical" and "horizontal" discourse to explore the significance of space and place in supervision. Data from a small qualitative study are used to illustrate the nuanced and complex nature in which issues of power and safety are navigated in supervision (Beddoe, 2011a).

Given that there is reported tendency for supervision to mirror the wider organisational climate (Davys & Beddoe, 2010) there is a concomitant need for education to promote reflective supervision to social workers at all levels (Bradley et al., 2010). Noble and Irwin (2009, p. 352) point out that it is not only managers who might promote less reflective styles of supervision, for new management practices require a "new kind of worker; a worker concerned with work performance and work appraisals, work outputs and management systems". From New Zealand, O'Donoghue (2012) reports how supervisors use their own experience of supervision as supervisees to guide their practice, confirming that practitioners' own supervision histories influence both positively and negatively on how they do supervision. In the commentary in 2012 we wrote that "the journey to becoming a supervisor is too often merely a rite of passage" without a formal, assessed period of education and training (Maidment & Beddoe, 2012, p. 165). In 2015 education for supervisors remains a priority within the profession and requires further research.

A further significant theme in the international literature addresses the retention of social workers in the workforce and their overall professional well-being. Self-defined resilient practitioners reported that supervision and team support were major contributing features of their sustained practice in social work (Beddoe, Davys & Adamson, 2014). Research on retention over the last decade has demonstrated links between effective supervision and social worker job satisfaction (Guerin, Devitt & Redmond, 2010) and well-being in the workplace (Kim & Lee, 2009; Mor Barak, Travis, Dnika, Pyun & Xie, 2009). In this current volume Chiller and Crisp report on the significance of supervision as an important contributing factor in the decisions of social workers to remain in practice for ten years or more. Practitioners most valued supervision for its "ability to act as a medium through which stresses and concerns can be externalised and explored" (Chiller & Crisp, 2012, p. 436). Adamson (2012) critically examines the resilience concept and argues that this discourse, focusing on the management of emotions, may provide the means for practitioners to negotiate the conflicting agendas of addressing risk, compliance and critical reflection in supervision.

Field Education

The future shape of field education supervision (practice teaching in some countries) is another area for potential development and significant change. Fostering quality learning and being mindful of resource management issues in field education are critical questions in the current milieu. A recent Australian study explored the use of external supervision for students in agencies where no qualified supervisor was present (Zuchowski, 2013). Increasingly accessing quality placements with on-site field educators has become difficult due to resource constraints within agencies and greater competition amongst education providers for placements. Findings from this study illustrated that students did not have a preference for internal or external supervision, despite the fact that external supervision was somehow perceived by students as being less desirable. Instead, the degree to which supervisors were prepared for having students, were able to provide the knowledge needed for practice and could provide support during the placement was seen as more important to students, than where the supervision was sited. (Zuchowski, 2013).

The quality of learning for Australian Aboriginal and Torres Strait Island students on placement and in supervision has been significantly challenged in findings from a second recent piece of Australian social work research (Zuchowski, Savage, Miles & Gair, 2013). Of significant concern in these separate Australian studies was overt racism being demonstrated towards clients and students by practitioners in placement agencies; bullying towards students; and less than optimal learning occurring due to both racist and sexist supervisor attitudes (Zuchowski et al., 2013; Zuchowski, 2013). Recommendations put forward by the authors suggest the urgent need for Indigenous mentors and supervisors in the workplace; acceptance and acknowledgement of different forms of knowledge for practice; and "increasing the cultural awareness and competence of staff in placement agencies and universities" (Zuchowski et al., 2013, p. 59). The serious lack of cultural competence and sensitivity amongst both staff in the agencies, including field supervisors, in this particular research is of significant concern to the profession. These worrying findings clearly demonstrate how Standard 3 of the Australian Association of Social Work Standards of Practice (2013), that of "Culturally responsive and inclusive practice" was not met by practitioners in the agencies where students were placed, and in some cases by the student supervisor themselves.

Culture in Supervision

While the literature cited above relates to a very specific context, the impact of culture on supervision relationships and effectiveness is an international concern. In light of the above research the development of cultural competence anti-oppressive practice in supervision in social work clearly continues to be of major importance for research and practice development. In 2009 Hair and O'Donoghue (p.74) challenged supervision authors and researchers to be more aware of culture stating that "leading social work supervision texts offer little to inform or encourage supervisors to integrate cultural knowledge" within their supervision practice. While there have been contributions on cross-cultural issues in supervision literature in general (see for example, De Souza, 2007; Hernández, Taylor & McDowell, 2009; Crocket, Flanagan, Alford, Allen, Baird et al., 2013) there is undoubtedly more work to do to support the inclusion of indigenous approaches into the supervision body of knowledge as the recent Australian research reported above attests. Research and development of indigenous approaches to supervision, such as the work of Eruera (2012) in Aotearoa New Zealand continues and the new body of knowledge on cultural models of supervision will continue to develop to enrich future supervision participants.

Hernández and McDowell (2010, p. 29) have urged supervisors to "prepare themselves to engage in critical analysis of dynamics of power" and to demonstrate "critical social awareness and cultural humility" in order to build effective supervision relationships. Supervision is not immune to changes brought about by globalisation and the internationalisation of social work education and practice, and social workers are increasingly involved in the business of supporting social, economic and cultural sustainability, as well as promoting humanitarian initiatives in response to crises. These concerns necessitate involvement with practice on national and global fronts, with supervision content and means of delivery needing to accommodate these changing conditions. Tsui, O'Donoghue and Ng (2014) have recently provided a valuable resource in reviewing the current literature on cross-cultural supervision to discover research and scholarship in this important field.

Where Next for Social Work Supervision?

O'Donoghue and Tsui (2013) have recently reported on a comprehensive review of supervision research articles published across the forty years from 1970 to 2010. This is an important review which has, according to the authors, demonstrated that: much of the research has been "derived from retrospective experiences of supervision"; research methods have "become more rigorous and diverse" and importantly that the research "provides a theory about social work supervision and what is thought to be good or not good, rather than empirically supported practice models" (O'Donoghue & Tsui, 2013, p. 13).

Echoing Carpenter, Webb, Bostock and Coomber (2012), O'Donoghue and Tsui suggest that what is needed is for research to focus on evaluating the effectiveness of supervision and develop "empirically supported supervision models"; explore how supervision "contributes to client outcomes and involve clients in supervision research"; and develop an international understanding of the nature and practice of supervision (2013, p. 13). As the editors of this collection we have given consideration to the potential "future agenda" for social work supervision and along with sharing these aims we believe that supervision research can usefully develop our understanding of practitioner well-being. Social work is by nature a demanding profession, with professional and organisational pressures adding to the toll of potentially corrosive exposure to stress (Van Heugten, 2011). Recent research by Adamson, Beddoe and Davys (2013) has explored practitioner understandings of resilience as a concept grounded not only in individual factors but influenced by workplace dynamics and organisational climate. Supervision has been identified by practitioners as a mechanism to help them remain resilient and hopeful in their practice (Adamson, 2012; Beddoe, Davys & Adamson, 2014; Collins, 2007) but disquiet regarding the mixing of line management and professional supervision is evident (Adamson, 2012; Beddoe, 2011a; Egan, 2012), while questions regarding the efficacy of external supervision arrangements have been canvassed (Cleak & Smith, 2012; Beddoe, 2011a). These concerns warrant further investment of time and effort to clarify and strengthen a distinction in practice, between line management supervision and professional supervision, focussed on fostering reflective practice in personal professional development. Such a division would result in functions relating to compliance, day-to-day case planning and risk management being addressed in a more explicit case management forum.

Functions related to critical reflection, professional knowledge building and systematic inquiry could be addressed in a forum such as "professional advancement". Reframing supervision functions in this way promotes transparency where line management tasks are separated out from forms of critical inquiry and professional development. While there has been significant attention to the role of reflection in social work supervision (Franklin, 2011; Bradbury-Jones, 2013) the process of encouraging forms of systematic inquiry and critical thinking within supervision have received less attention. The functions of critical inquiry and knowledge building could take place in a forum for "professional advancement", a type of group supervision and learning space where conversations about evidence based practice and advanced professional development topics could occur. In this era where evidence based practice has such purchase for attracting funding and providing justification for programing decisions (Gilgun, 2005), practitioners need a forum to engage in research informed practice discussions. Little has been written about the extent to which discussions about research occur in traditional supervision, yet it is well known that social workers are not confident in their interpretations of research or in conducting practice research themselves (Beddoe, 2011b). Nevertheless, competence to engage with research is necessary at the practitioner level where resource allocation is increasingly based on proven effectiveness of service delivery.

We believe it is time to make space to introduce discussions about research into supervision, whether this occurs on an individual or group basis. Ideally these conversations would happen in both student and practitioner supervision or advanced professional forums as discussed above. A starting point could be to source a couple of research articles about the relevant field of practice for both supervisor and supervisee to read in preparation for the next supervision session. Select from the articles points of interest, areas not understood or ideas for future practice, and make these the basis for beginning a conversation about the relationship between research and service delivery. We have noted the paucity of literature on the ways research is incorporated into social work supervision, suggesting a need for this topic, in and of itself, to become a focus for future disciplinary research.

The research and scholarship presented in this volume, considered alongside the literature which has emerged since the publication of the special issue in 2012, suggests that supervision scholarship is in good heart. There is a need for further research, and the reviews conducted by Carpenter and colleagues (Carpenter, Webb, Bostock & Coomber, 2012; Carpenter, Webb & Bostock, 2013) and O'Donoghue and Tsui (2013) have provided an important overview with a map of suggested ways forward. A pertinent challenge to supervision researchers is to look beyond one-to-one transaction supervision models and seek to explore models that can revitalise group and peer approaches. In these times of constrained budgets and downsizing we need as a profession to find ways to resource professional development, while still attending to individual practitioner needs for revitalisation and support, without undue financial burden to the agency or individual practitioners. We hope that colleagues in practice and academia will pick up the challenge to explore the potential for new models so that supervision may continue to respond to professional needs and workplace complexities.

References

Adamson, C. (2012). Supervision is not politically innocent. *Australian Social Work, 65*(2), 185–196. doi:10.1080/0312407x.2011.618544

Australian Association of Social Work (2013). *Practice Standards.* http://www.aasw.asn.au/document/item/4551

Baines, D., Charlesworth, S., Turner, D., & O'Neill, L. (2014). Lean social care and worker identity: The role of outcomes, supervision and mission. *Critical Social Policy.* doi:10.1177/0261018314538799

Beddoe, L. (2010). Surveillance or reflection: Professional supervision in 'the risk society'. *British Journal of Social Work, 40*(4), 1279–1296. doi:10.1093/bjsw/bcq018

Beddoe, L. (2011a). External supervision in social work: Power, space, risk, and the search for safety. *Australian Social Work, 65*(2), 197–213. doi:10.1080/0312407x.2011.591187

Beddoe, L. (2011b). Investing in the future: Social workers talk about research. *British Journal of Social Work, 41*(3), 557–575. doi:10.1093/bjsw/bcq138

Beddoe, L., Davys, A. M., & Adamson, C. (2014). 'Never trust anybody who says "I don't need supervision"': Practitioners' beliefs about social worker resilience. *Practice, 26*(2), 113–130. doi:10.1080/09503153.2014.896888

Bradbury-Jones, C. (2013) Refocusing child protection supervision: An innovative approach to supporting practitioners. *Child Care in Practice, 19*(3), 253–266. doi:10.1080/13575279.2013.785937

Bradley, G., & Höjer, S. (2009). Supervision reviewed: reflections on two different social work models in England and Sweden. *European Journal of Social Work, 12*(1), 71–85.

Bradley, G., Engelbrecht, L., & Höjer, S. (2010). Supervision: A force for change? Three stories told. *International Social Work, 53*(6), 773–790.

Carpenter, J., Webb, C. M., Bostock, L., & Coomber, C. (2012). Effective supervision in social work and social care. *Research Briefing 43.* London: Social Care Institute for Excellence.

Carpenter, J., Webb, C. M., & Bostock, L. (2013). The surprisingly weak evidence base for supervision: Findings from a systematic review of research in child welfare practice (2000–2012). *Children and Youth Services Review, 35*(11), 1843–1853. doi: http://dx.doi.org/10.1016/j.childyouth.2013.08.014

Chiller, P., & Crisp, B. R. (2012). Professional supervision: A workforce retention strategy for social work? *Australian Social Work, 65*(2), 232–242. doi:10.1080/0312407x.2011.625036

Cleak, H., & Smith, D. (2012). Student satisfaction with models of field placement supervision. *Australian Social Work, 65*(2), 243–258. doi:10.1080/0312407x.2011.572981

Collins, S. (2007). Social workers, resilience, positive emotions and optimism. *Practice, 19*(4), 255–269.

Crocket, K., Flanagan, P., Alford, Z., Allen, J., Baird, J., Bruce, A., Swann, H. (2013). Supervision and culture: Meetings at thresholds. *New Zealand Journal of Counselling 33*(1), 68–86.

Davys, A., & Beddoe, L. (2010). *Best practice in supervision: A guide for the helping professions.* London: Jessica Kingsley.

De Souza, R. (2007). Multicultural relationships in supervision. In D. Wepa (Ed.), *Clinical supervision in Aotearoa/New Zealand: A health perspective* (pp. 96–108). Auckland: Pearson Education.

Egan, R. (2012). Australian social work supervision practice in 2007. *Australian Social Work, 65*(2), 171–184. doi:10.1080/0312407x.2011.653575

Eruera, M. (2012). He kōrari, he kete, he korero. *Aotearoa New Zealand Social Work Review, 24*(3/4), 12–19.

Franklin, L. (2011). Reflective supervision for the green social worker: Practical applications for supervisors. *Clinical Supervisor, 30*(2), 204–214. doi:10.1080/07325223.2011.607743

Gilgun, J. (2005). The four cornerstones of evidence-based practice in social work. *Research on Social Work Practice. 15*(22), 52–61.

Guerin, S., Devitt, C., & Redmond, B. (2010). Experiences of early-career social workers in Ireland. *British Journal of Social Work, 40*(8), 2467–2484. doi:10.1093/bjsw/bcq020

Hair, H. J. (2013). The purpose and duration of supervision, and the training and discipline of supervisors: What social workers say they need to provide effective services. *British Journal of Social Work, 43*(8), 1562–1588. doi:10.1093/bjsw/bcs071

Hair, H. J. (2014a). Power relations in supervision: Preferred practices according to social workers. *Families in Society: The Journal of Contemporary Social Services, 95*(2), 107–114.

Hair, H. J. (2014b). Supervision conversations about social justice and social work practice. *Journal of Social Work.* doi:10.1177/1468017314539082

Hair, H. J., & O'Donoghue, K. (2009). Culturally relevant, socially just social work supervision: Becoming visible through a social constructionist lens. *Journal of Ethnic and Cultural Diversity in Social Work, 18*(1), 70–88.

Hernández, P., Taylor, B., & McDowell, T. (2009). Listening to ethnic minority AAMFT approved supervisors: Reflections on their experiences as supervisees. *Journal of Systemic Therapies, 28*(1), 88.

Hernández, P., & McDowell, T. (2010). Intersectionality, power, and relational safety in context: Key concepts in clinical supervision. *Training and Education in Professional Psychology, 4*(1), 29–35. doi: 10.1037/a0017064

Jones, M. (2004). Supervision, learning and transformative practices. In N. Gould & M. Baldwin (Eds.), *Social work, critical reflection and the learning organisation* (pp. 11–22). Aldershot: Ashgate.

Kim, H., & Lee, S. Y. (2009). Supervisory communication, burnout, and turnover intention among social workers in health care settings. *Social Work in Health Care, 48*(4), 364–385.

Maidment, J., & Beddoe, L. (2012). Is social work supervision in "good heart"? A critical commentary. *Australian Social Work, 65*(2), 163–170. doi:10.1080/0312407x.2012.680426

Morrison, T. (2001). *Staff supervision in social care: Making a real difference for staff and service users.* Brighton: Pavilion.

Mor Barak, M. E., Travis, DnikaJ., Pyun, H., & Xie, B. (2009). The impact of supervision on worker outcomes: A meta-analysis. *Social Service Review, 83*(1), 3–32. doi:10.1086/599028

Noble, C., & Irwin, J. (2009). Social work supervision: An exploration of the current challenges in a rapidly changing social, economic and political environment. *Journal of Social Work, 9*(3), 345–358. doi:10.1177/1468017309334848

O'Donoghue, K. (2012). Windows on the supervisee experience: An exploration of supervisees' supervision histories. *Australian Social Work, 65*(2), 214–231. doi:10.1080/0312407x.2012.667816

O'Donoghue, K., & Tsui, M.-s. (2013). Social work supervision research (1970–2010): The way we were and the way ahead. *British Journal of Social Work.* doi:10.1093/bjsw/bct115

Richards, M., & Payne, C. (1991). *Staff supervision in child protection work.* London: National Institute for Social Work.

Tsui, M.-s., O'Donoghue, K., & Ng, A. K. T. (2014). Culturally competent and diversity-sensitive clinical supervision. In C. E. Watkins, Jr., & D. L. Milne (Eds.), *The Wiley International Handbook of Clinical Supervision* (pp. 238–254). Chichester: John Wiley & Sons, Ltd.

Van Heugten, K. (2011). *Social Work under Pressure.* London: Jessica Kingsley.

Zuchowski, I. (2013). From being 'caught in the middle of a war' to being 'in a really safe space' – social work field education with external supervision. *Advances in Social Work and Welfare Education, 15*(1), 104–120.

Zuchowski, I., Savage, D., Miles, D., & Gair, S. (2013). Decolonising field education: Challenging Australian social work praxis. *Advances in Social Work and Welfare Education, 15*(1), 47–62.

Supervision is Not Politically Innocent

Carole Adamson

School of Counselling, Human Services & Social Work, University of Auckland, Auckland, New Zealand

Abstract

This paper argues that the potential tensions within the role, function, and purpose of supervision, potentially magnified by the adoption of the process within a variety of organisational and occupational settings, underscore the importance of supervision being seen as a contextually informed activity. Supervision can be constructed as a professional development activity with processes of reflection that are potentially active contributors to practitioner resilience. It can also be viewed as a developmental tool that assists a worker adapt to the workplace context and to process environmentally located challenges and tensions. Within some workplaces, supervision has an active managerial and risk-management function. Using the lens of resilience theories, this paper addresses key issues for supervision emerging from its different functions and argues that in becoming aware of its contextual location in complex practice and organisational environments, supervision practice itself cannot remain politically innocent.

The practice of supervision in professional contexts has extended beyond social work and into health and human services, education, counselling, and psychotherapy (Davys & Beddoe, 2010). Much of the supervision literature has focused upon the quality of the supervisory relationship (Tsui, 2005); issues for implementing supervision for different disciplines (Davys & Beddoe, 2009); and variations in the delivery of supervision in the light of technological and geographical imperatives such as practice in remote areas of Australia (Lonne & Cheers, 2004), online supervision (Allan, Crockett, Ball, Alston, & Whittenbury, 2007), interdisciplinary accountabilities (Bogo, Paterson, Tufford, & King, 2011; Davys & Beddoe, 2009; Townend, 2005) and so forth. A broad distinction between "micro" and "macro" issues has emerged, with much "micro" focus upon what could be constructed as intra- and interpersonal concerns, the ethics of relationships, and quality-control issues of best practice. This paper offers a contribution to the "macro" focus of supervision practice, workforce, and organisational concerns by addressing the centrality of the contextual dynamics of supervision. Using concepts from resilience literature, the paper argues that supervision within social work is not a politically or organisationally neutral practice but one that must be constantly aware of its context, purpose, and application. In so being, it suggests that the relationship between the practice of supervision and the values and identity of social work can remain vibrant.

Practising Supervision in Context

Supervision never happens in a vacuum. The extension of the role and function of professional supervision throughout and beyond social work has magnified our understanding of the competing tensions that it contains, as different occupational groupings seek to adapt and interpret supervision to meet their specific needs and contexts. Social work literature itself attests to the multiplicity of purposes to which this relational, occupational process can be put.

Early conceptualisations, such as that of Kadushin (1992), identified the potential synergies or disruptions between administrative, education, and supportive functions. Unpacking this further, Kadushin's categories introduced notions of accountability, policies, procedures, and standards; acquisition and expansion of knowledge and skills; and maintenance and strengthening of morale and job satisfaction. Adoption of supervision as a tool for nonmanagerial purposes has led to a growth in understanding about supervision as a professional or consultative, quality enhancement activity that intertwines practitioner reflection and growth with best practice notions of effective clinical skills and positive therapeutic outcomes for clients (Bernard & Goodyear, 1992).

This produces a potentially conflicting range of possible roles, functions, and purposes for supervision, all of which will play out within the various organisational and political environments in which professional practice is supervised. These often competing tensions, highlighted by Hawkins and Shohet (1989) and Beddoe (2010), can be depicted as a "swingometer" (adapted from Chapman's concept, initially applied to election forecasting and described in Easton, 2003) whose pendulum falls at various points between a focus on practice competence and on accountability, dependent upon practitioner or management interpretation or upon policy demands of resource allocation or risk assessment.

On the left of the framework are the professional concerns of practitioner expertise, capturing some of the educational and support functions that Kadushin described, along with developmental notions such as Hawkins and Shohet's (1989) transition from self-centred to process-in-context practitioner and Butler's (1996) development of the practitioner from novice to expert. The emphasis here is on reflective capacity and professional development, which is in harmony with the attention to quality, best practice, and consumer and client rights that can generally be described as having a clinical focus (Bernard & Goodyear, 1992; Feltham & Dryden, 1994; Goldhammer, Anderson, & Krajewski, 1993; Howard, 2008; Tsui, 2005). Overall, these two functions described at the left of the diagram focus on the

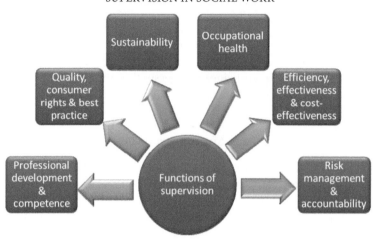

Figure 1 The supervision "swingometer"

relational aspects of the practitioner and the client, embedding their connection within the specifics of the service provided.

The area where the work of Kadushin and these other, relatively early, writers is perhaps the least developed occurs where the pendulum swings further to the right. It first encounters issues of sustainability of practice and of occupational health. It is here that the writings of Brown and Bourne (1996) are widely used in the teaching of supervision practice, as they more actively embed supervision as a practice within an agency context and construct the supervision journey as a development process from induction to connection and on into integration. New social workers progressively develop understandings about their role, the client's world, the team, the agency, and the bigger contextual issues. Issues of resilience and stress are employed in this perspective on supervision, with a person-in-environment recognition of the impact of the work on the worker (Collins, 2007).

The right-hand domains towards which the pendulum can swing describe the activities and purposes of supervision that are determined by managerial require-ments, organisationally determined outcomes that are perhaps normative in nature, with a potential to become focused on public accountability within a risk-averse political environment (Beddoe, 2010). These demands upon the supervision process place emphasis on the organisational (as opposed to the clinical, client-focused, or professional) activities and responsibilities of the social worker and are a trend observed in social work supervision by Adams (2007). Collins (2007) referred to the earlier work of Gorman (2000) and Rogers (2001), both of whom suggested that the focus on cost-effectiveness and efficiency reduces a focus on the relational and emotional content of social work. From a constructionist perspective, Hair and O'Donoghue (2009) suggested that this interpretation of the role stems from a modernist construction of supervisor-as-expert and serves to ignore the wider social and political contexts in which supervision occurs. Supervision occurring within these environments may have the most apparent tensions as supervisors and supervisees grapple with the balance between clinical, professional, and managerial accountabilities.

Acknowledgement of these different and potentially competing functions of supervision is, of course, one that is actively negotiated within the construction of supervision contracts and managed skilfully within many supervision settings (Jones, 2004). Supervisors and supervisees constantly juggle performance review functions with support and professional development activities. The argument of this paper is that, once these tensions are recognised, the contextual location of supervision and the resulting dynamics (those that are termed "political" in this paper) cannot be ignored. With this, the imperative to balance risk management with practitioner reflection and development perspectives becomes crucial. It is suggested here that the use of a resilience lens can assist practitioners and supervisors to negotiate this territory.

Using the Lens of Resilience

Arguably, there is no unique theory of resilience as applied to client groups or to ourselves as practitioners. We can chart the evolution of concepts of resiliency from an early focus on pathology, intrapsychic and individual strengths, where both the causes and the solutions to stressors lie within the individual's personality, skills, and re-sources (Cederblad & Dahlin, 1995). The evolution proceeds through the ascendancy of systems theories (Lewis, 2000) and a greater relational, ecological, or contextual awareness of the power of the environment to determine or limit opportunity (Garmezy, Masten, & Tellegen, 1984; Mackay, 2003) to a current understanding that both individual and collective narratives can interplay with broad community-level and structural factors to create diverse patterns of coping and resilience (Bottrell, 2009; Ungar, 2004, 2008). Such transitions reflect the developments in western perspectives in human services and in social work, where we can trace the shift from pathogenic to salutogenic approaches (Antonovsky, 1996; Bottrell, 2009; Eriksson & Lindström, 2008; van Breda, 2011); from psychodynamic to constructivist constructs; and from reductionist to holistic and strengths perspectives.

Therefore, the development of the concept of resilience for social work has an evolution from a focus on individual characteristics to a greater awareness of contextual and environmental influence and interaction (Bottrell, 2009). Resilience is not currently constructed as dependent upon one dominant factor, but rather as the activation and interaction of an array of possible resources both internal and external to the person.

The importance of tracking this change in the manner in which we understand human strengths and coping mechanisms can be summed up by stating that current conceptualisation of the factors that create resilience recognises that a person becomes resilient through an interplay of individual, relational, systemic, and structural factors that flex and flux over time and place. Luthar and Cicchetti (2000) conceptualised resilience as an adaptive process. This enables a definition of resilience to move from construction as the ability to bounce back from events of adversity to a

13

consideration of a matrix of factors that build the ability to withstand pressure and adapt over time. The development of strengths approaches allows for the description of protective factors that can shield a person or mediate with the environment to lessen the impact of adversity or cumulative pressure. This interactive model can add weight to our understanding of supervision in context.

Collins (2007) suggested that most of the resilience literature has focused on children, with less attention paid to adults. In addition, a small but growing body of research and literature has turned the spotlight of resilience from the "other" (the client) towards the worker in a social work context or system (Russ, Lonne, & Darlington, 2009; van Breda, 2011). It can be argued that this relative paucity of literature is an artefact of the transitional status of the concepts of stress and resilience that continue to move away from a pathological stance (identifying the "problems" in the objects of social worker attention, i.e., clients) towards an interactive and more relational construction of wellness and coping that turns the spotlight equally on the self of the worker. Considerably more literature exists concerning the negative impact of our practice, vicarious and secondary traumatisation, and burnout. There has been less of a specific emphasis on the positive relationship between social work practice and the ameliorative contribution of supervision to the maintenance of best practice and the resilience of the social worker, although some strong studies are now coming through (Collins, 2007; Kinman & Grant, 2011; Mor Barak, Travis, Pyun, & Xie, 2009). While some key arguments can be drawn from this literature, there remains considerable scope to tease out some principles from the resilience literature focused on the "other" and apply them to the workplace and the supervision context. Thus, questions of the correlation and goodness of fit between these principles and supervision provide rich territory for supervision-specific resilience research.

What then can we take from an understanding of resilience that applies to supervision in diverse social work contexts? How does this knowledge guide our awareness of supervision as a contested, political activity with a multiplicity of roles and functions? Using the resilience literature to inform the discussion, this paper tracks the pendulum of the swingometer from consideration of supervision as a reflective tool, focusing upon professional and clinical development and relational expertise that results in effective practice, through a focus upon the sustainability and wellbeing of the workforce, to a consideration of employer and organisational interests in the concept of resilience. In so doing, key issues concerning the link between resilience and supervision in complex environments will be considered.

Supervision in Relation to Professional Development and Best Practice

"Reflection for Resilience"

Current perspectives have suggested that the resilience of an individual at any given time will be a dynamic response to both risk and resiliency factors that brings together their personal history and current environmental demands (Bonanno, Westphal, & Mancini, 2011). With no one universal or dominant characteristic determining hardiness in the face of adversity, this paper suggests that there is potential for supervision to provide a healthy environment for strengthening the professional development and best practice of the supervisee, the left-hand components of the framework. A core element of this function of supervision is that of reflection.

To "take something to supervision" is a term that often refers to the process of creating space within a supervision session in order to address a complex, multi-stranded situation. The process of responding to what Butler, Ford, and Tregaskis (2007) termed "the messy complexities of practice" (p. 285) is the process of reflection, a term that Noble (1999) described as linking the thinking and the doing, and the doing and the thinking. A key role of supervision in social work is the strengthening of a worker's ability to respond to uncertainty and complexity (Askeland & Fook, 2009; Burgess, 2004; Lymbery, 2003; Parton, 1998). The Australian Association of Social Workers [AASW] Education and Accreditation Standards (e.g., AASW, 2008) acknowledged that complex practice situations are responded to by attention to reflective and reflexive practice, structural analysis, critical thinking, and ethical professional behaviour. The notion of "seeing the wood for the trees", of ascertaining what is personal, professional, or political, is core to the supervision process. It is within this space that we explore uncertainty and develop narratives and alternative possibilities.

The relevance of a resilience knowledgebase to this function of supervision is, as Howe (2008) suggested, that the management of emotions underpins resilience. From a psychologically informed theory of resilience, supervision can be constructed as an opportunity for positive reappraisal of complex situations and one's own emotional responses. Collins (2007) constructed supervision as a protective process, with emotional knowledge and positive emotions building up emotional regulation and trait resilience. Referring to Nathan (1993), Collins described reflective thinking as transforming emotional chaos into containable anxiety. Kinman and Grant (2011) suggested that emotional intelligence and aspects of empathy and social competence may be key protective qualities, with reflective ability being "an important predictor of resilience and psychological well-being" (p. 10).

A key strand of reflection for resilience emerges as support for the maintenance and growth of optimism and hope (Collins, 2007; Schwartz, Tiamiyu, & Dwyer, 2007). Similarly, Kinman and Grant (2011) and Morrison (2007) addressed the development of emotional and social competencies, while Stalker, Mandell, Frensch, Harvey, and Wright (2007) considered factors that enable exhausted social workers to maintain satisfaction in their work. Therefore, supervision, as a site for creating a reflective and mediating space for the consideration and comprehension of the emotional impact of experience, can be strongly supported as a process that can maintain and sustain resilience.

With a focus upon the professional functions of supervision, the left-hand side of the swingometer, the synergy between social work values and perspectives with the knowledgebase of resilience appears relatively congruent. Supervision, constructed as a reflective space and activity, is unproblematically linked with supporting resilience in social work. Where the pendulum moves towards workforce (as opposed to practice-focused) functions and managerial need, the relationship with a resilience knowledgebase, although remaining strong, becomes more contestable.

Supervision's Contribution Towards Sustaining and Maintaining the Workforce

Previously in this paper, the developmental models of Hawkins and Shohet (1989), Butler (1996), and of Brown and Bourne (1996) have been acknowledged as being significant to shaping our understanding of the supervision relationship as a developmental process, locating the exploration of these issues within the "sustainability of practice" and "occupational health" foci of the swingometer. These models recognise that the supervisee moves through stages (often sequentially but never perhaps fluidly or directionally consistently) from a beginner in induction through to a practitioner with more highly developed levels of competence and integration. Increasingly, this perspective has incorporated comprehension that it is the supervisory relationship itself that undergoes development (e.g., Kadushin & Harkness, 2002), albeit not without issues of an imbalance of power (Cooper, 2002; Noble & Irwin, 2009).

From both the supervision and resilience literature (Bottrell, 2009; Brown & Bourne, 1996) comes the argument that the environment has a considerable role in facilitating the development of a person in an organisational and supervision context. Attachment theory, relational to its core, informs both supervision and resilience. Bennett (2008) suggested that both embedded and newly created patterns of attachment may determine the outcome of supervisory relationships within the workplace environment. It is the acknowledgement of supervision as a developmental process within a complex and demanding work environment that shifts the use of resilience theory away from a simple interpretation of the importance of reflection to a more critical role of developing reflexive practice and contextual strategies for coping.

There is emerging evidence in the literature that supervision has a crucial role in the wellbeing of early-career social workers (Guerin, Devitt, & Redmond, 2010). Jack and Donnellan (2010) suggested that it is the neglect of the development of social workers through a focus upon knowledge and task completion that erodes their capacity to thrive in complex and demanding roles.

Mor Barak et al. (2009) argued that "effective supervision at the worker's level can contribute to such positive worker outcomes as job satisfaction, organizational commitment, and worker retention" (p. 4). Their meta-analysis considered that effective supervision "is known to serve as a buffer against stressful work conditions, to provide protection from unreasonable job demands, to offer emotional and social support during difficult times, and to guide workers in negotiating the challenges of the job and the organizational context" (p. 4). They suggested that there is organisational benefit in constructing policies and enabling resources focused upon positive supervision relationships and stress the importance of organisational culture and strengthen the case for structuring reflective and reflexive practice as foundations for resilience.

Studies of the resilience of client groups have highlighted a further potential application of theories of resilience to supervision and the wellbeing of social workers. Bottrell (2009) suggested that social and environmental barriers (processes or structures) may inhibit optimal development. While researching young people within a low-income urban environment in Sydney, she found that positive outcomes were impeded or prevented by rigid structures, perceptions, and poor relationships between resources and communities. Applying this notion of resilience to the supervision relationship within an organisational context, barriers to optimum development may take the form of inadequate induction or orientation procedures; lack of clarity in roles and responsibilities; a poor fit with cultural expectations; interdisciplinary confusions or rivalries, and so forth. Whether the barriers are individual, relational, cultural, systemic, or structural, unsuccessful negotiation may result in poor performance and an erosion of the quality of the supervision relationship itself. Supervision's embedded position within the relational dynamics of an organisation necessitates acknowledgement of how barriers such as these may affect development and outcome.

A resilience lens underscores the importance of the relational, both within and external to the supervision relationship. Current concepts of resilience are predicated upon the fundamental assumption that social support is one of the main buffers against stress. For instance, Collins (2007) reflected upon how a team of social workers can provide a protective environment and argued that changes in personnel and management can produce vulnerability for individuals within the system. Supervision needs to be cognisant of relationships and structurally determined patterns of communication external to, as well as within, the supervision. A robust supervision relationship can act as a resilience buffer in a less-than-optimum working environment; similarly, a poor relationship may limit the development of, or access to, wider organisational knowledge or resources.

With the resilience concept of barriers to development comes the risk of normalising a person's behaviour or performance. If barriers are not recognised, the supervisee may be judged according to external norms or expectations. Their inadequate use of resources may be due to poor induction processes rather than to a lack of networking skills.

Our understanding of barriers to the development of resilience is complemented by notions of "hidden" resilience (Ungar, 2004, 2008). Here, supervisee resilience may not be as much impeded by environmental issues external to the person, as much as that they may possess attributes or demonstrate behaviours that either go unrecognised by others or are not recognised as strengths. Within social work, this may be exemplified by a young person missing school. The importance of their role in keeping the family together by caring for a sick parent or siblings may go unrecognised; they may be labelled according to external norms as "failing". Similarly, within the workplace someone whose skills or interests are mismatched with their role requirements may be adjudged a poor performer. For instance, workers selected for cultural expertise may consider their role in community development as taking priority over agency requirements and their behaviour judged as poor time-keeping, absenteeism, or a lack of commitment. A child protection worker may commit comparatively more time to one family, with a view to a therapeutic outcome, than agency targets permit.

Resilience literature cautions us against taking a normative stance in supervision. Bottrell (2009) and Ungar's (2004, 2008) presentation of personal, local, and cultural definitions suggested that a person's resilience can only be assessed through an understanding of their own perceptions, interactions, and contexts. We ignore personal or cultural narratives at our peril. Hair and O'Donoghue (2009) outlined the risks inherent in cultural assumptions within cross-cultural supervision, risks that include not only interpersonal "talking past each other" but assumptions about the process of relationship, culturally specific systems of support, or the structures of supervision delivery compatible within and across cultures or organisational settings.

Noble and Irwin (2009) reflected upon the trend to try out different forms of supervision within social work, considering that this was a result of the managerial and accountability focus of the traditional model of one-to-one supervision and was a demonstration of social workers attempting to move the focus of the process back from organisational demands towards attention to professional practice (the left-hand side of the swingometer). In this way, supervision may become a site of resistance. It is to the issues that confront supervision on the right-hand side of the framework that the discussion now turns.

Implications of Applying Resiliency Theory to Supervision

Resilience in Adverse Environments

Resilience is often defined as an ability to withstand adversity. Within environments that have an undue measure of adverse conditions, the application of concepts of resilience is not without fish-hooks. Kinman and Grant (2011) suggested that "even the most resilient social workers will be unable to thrive under working conditions that are pathogenic" (p. 12). They suggested that this gives us the mandate to pay attention to the structural and systemic issues of social work roles beyond reactive, individualised self-care and stress-management strategies and instead place a focus upon wellbeing and salutogenic environments. From a focus on client resilience, Bottrell (2009) argued that a contextually aware definition of resilience requires us to focus upon bigger picture issues (the "political") of policy demands, competing interests, and organisational conditions. Indeed, it can be argued that a capacity to see the bigger picture and to put issues within a context is in itself a factor that can contribute to resilience.

Matching these core tenets of current resiliency theory to social work values illustrates that, for practitioners, there is an ethical and political imperative to place a spotlight on inequitable conditions for both clients and colleagues. In applying concepts of resilience within supervision, it follows that indicators of stress, inequality, or injustice explored within the supervision relationship also become matters for consideration and ethical inquiry. Beddoe (2010) and Jones (2004) both argued that the construction of the supervisory role will be porous to the social and political tensions in its wider environment. In organisational settings that are risk-sensitive and which have a strong focus on managerial accountabilities, resilience theories within supervision may be applied for purposes of performance management and damage limitation. The construction of a person or team as resilient suggests that key resources may be relocated to apparently more problematic areas with a view to reducing organisational exposure to risk. Being seen to cope may mean being left without the resources with which to do the job, or may entail being given so much more work that competence is threatened. A measurement of competence—such an environmentally sensitive capacity—could potentially erode, rather than strengthen, support.

Conclusion

In conclusion, then, how much adversity should a social worker cope with? There may be risks associated with the adoption of resilience theories without contextual and political awareness. Bottrell (2009) suggested that "resilience building in a neoliberal framework may shift the emphasis from positive adaptation despite adversity to positive adaptation *to* adversity" (p. 334). The conditions that determine resilience may be located outside of the individual social work practitioner and their professional development, supervision relationship, or team. If so, the theories that social work uses to support the provision of supervision (and indeed, the arguments for supervision itself) must be acutely mindful of the contexts in which they are applied. Supervision is not, and should never be presumed to be, politically innocent.

References

Adams, J. (2007). *Managing people in organisations: Contemporary theory and practice.* Basingstoke, UK: Palgrave Macmillan.

Allan, J., Crockett, J., Ball, P., Alston, M., & Whittenbury, K. (2007). 'It's all part of the package' in rural allied health: A pilot study of rewards and barriers in rural pharmacy and social work. *The Internet Journal of Allied Health Sciences and Practice, 5* (3).

Antonovsky, A. (1996). The salutogenic model as a theory to guide health promotion. *Health Promotion International, 11* (1), 11–18.

Askeland, G. A., & Fook, J. (2009). Critical reflection in social work. *European Journal of Social Work, 12* (3), 287–292.

Australian Association of Social Workers [AASW]. (2008). *Australian social work education and accreditation standards.* Canberra, ACT: Australian Association of Social Workers.

Beddoe, L. (2010). Surveillance or reflection: Professional supervision in "the risk society". *British Journal of Social Work, 40* (4), 1279–1296.

Bennett, C. S. (2008). Attachment-informed supervision for social work field education. *Clinical Social Work, 36* (1), 97–107.

Bernard, J. M., & Goodyear, R. K. (1992). Fundamentals of clinical supervision. Boston, MA: Allyn & Bacon.

Bogo, M., Paterson, J., Tufford, L., & King, R. (2011). Interprofessional clinical supervision in mental health and addiction: Toward identifying common elements. *The Clinical Supervisor, 30* (1), 124–140.

Bonanno, G. A., Westphal, M., & Mancini, A. D. (2011). Resilience to loss and potential trauma. *Annual Review of Clinical Psychology, 7* (1), 511–535.

Bottrell, D. (2009). Understanding "marginal" perspectives: Towards a social theory of resilience. *Qualitative Social Work, 8,* 321–339.

Brown, A., & Bourne, I. (1996). *The social work supervisor: Supervision in community, daycare and residential settings.* Buckingham, UK: Open University Press.

Burgess, H. (2004). Redesigning the curriculum for social work education: Complexity, conformity, chaos, creativity, collaboration? *Social Work Education, 23* (2), 163–183.

Butler, J. (1996). Professional development: Practice as text, reflection as process, and self as locus. *Australian Journal of Education, 40* (3), 265–283.

Butler, A., Ford, D., & Tregaskis, C. (2007). Who do we think we are? Self and reflexivity in social work practice. *Qualitative Social Work, 6* (3), 281–299.

Cederblad, M., & Dahlin, L. (1995). Intelligence and temperament as protective factors for mental health: A cross-sectional and prospective epidemiology study. *European Archives of Psychiatry and Clinical Neuroscience, 245,* 11–19.

Collins, S. (2007). Social workers, resilience, positive emotions and optimism. *Practice, 19* (4), 255–269.

Cooper, L. (2002). Social work supervision: A social justice perspective. In M. McMahon & W. Patton (Eds.), *Supervision in the helping professions: A practical approach* (pp. 185–195). Frenchs Forest, NSW: Pearson Australia.

Davys, A. M., & Beddoe, E. (2009). Interprofessional learning for supervision: "Taking the blinkers off". *Learning in Health and Social Care, 8* (1), 58–69.

Davys, A. M., & Beddoe, E. (2010). *Best practice in professional supervision: A guide for the helping professions.* London: Jessica Kingsley.

Easton, B. (2003). The political economy of Robert Chapman. *Political Science, 55* (1), 55–62.

Eriksson, M., & Lindström, B. (2008). A salutogenic interpretation of the Ottawa Charter. *Health Promotion International, 23* (2), 190–199.

Feltham, C., & Dryden, W. (1994). *Developing counsellor supervision.* London: Sage.

Garmezy, N., Masten, A. S., & Tellegen, A. (1984). The study of stress and competence in children: A building block for developmental psychopathology. *Child Development, 55* (1), 97–111.

Goldhammer, R., Anderson, R. H., & Krajewski, R. J. (1993). *Clinical supervision: Special methods for the supervision of teachers* (3rd ed.). Fort Worth, TX: Harcourt Brace Jovanovich.

Gorman, H. (2000). Winning hearts and minds? Emotional labour and learning for care management work. *Journal of Social Work Practice, 14* (2), 149–158.

Guerin, S., Devitt, C., & Redmond, B. (2010). Experiences of early-career social workers in Ireland. *British Journal of Social Work, 40* (8), 2467–2484.

Hair, H. J., & O'Donoghue, K. (2009). Culturally relevant, socially just social work supervision: Becoming visible through a social constructionist lens. *Journal of Ethnic and Cultural Diversity in Social Work, 18* (1), 70–88.

Hawkins, P., & Shohet, R. (1989). *Supervision in the helping professions.* Milton Keynes, UK: Open University Press.

Howard, F. (2008). Managing stress or enhancing wellbeing? Positive psychology's contributions to clinical supervision. *Australian Psychologist, 43* (2), 105–113.

Howe, D. (2008). *The emotionally intelligent social worker.* London: Palgrave McMillan.

Jack, G., & Donnellan, H. (2010). Recognising the person within the developing professional: Tracking the early careers of newly qualified child care social workers in three local authorities in England. *Social Work Education, 29* (3), 305–318.

Jones, M. (2004). Supervision, learning and transformative practices. In N. Gould & M. Baldwin (Eds.), *Social work, critical reflection and the learning organisation* (pp. 11–22). Aldershot: Ashgate.

Kadushin, A. (1992). *Supervision in social work* (3rd ed.). New York: Columbia University Press.

Kadushin, A., & Harkness, D. (2002). *Supervision in social work* (4th ed.). New York: Columbia University Press.

Kinman, G., & Grant, L. (2011). Exploring stress resilience in trainee social workers: The role of emotional and social competencies. *British Journal of Social Work, 41* (2), 261–275.

Lewis, M. D. (2000). The promise of dynamic systems approaches for an integrated account of human development. *Child Development, 71* (1), 36–43.

Lonne, B., & Cheers, B. (2004). Retaining rural social workers: An Australian study. *Rural Society, 14* (2), 163–177.

Luthar, S., & Cicchetti, D. (2000). The construct of resilience: Implications for interventions and social policies. *Development and Psychopathology, 12,* 857–885.

Lymbery, M. (2003). Negotiating the contradictions between competence and creativity in social work education. *Journal of Social Work, 3* (1), 99–117.

Mackay, R. (2003). Family resilience and good child outcomes: An overview of the research literature. *Social Policy Journal of New Zealand, 20* (June), 98–118.

Mor Barak, M., Travis, D. J., Pyun, H., & Xie, B. (2009). The impact of supervision on worker outcomes: A meta-analysis. *Social Service Review, 83* (1), 3–32.

Morrison, T. (2007). Emotional intelligence, emotion, and social work: Context, characteristics, complications and contribution. *British Journal of Social Work, 37* (2), 245–263.

Nathan, J. (1993). The battered social worker: A psychodynamic contribution to practice, supervision and policy. *Journal of Social Work Practice, 7* (1), 73–80.

Noble, C. (1999). The elusive yet essential project of developing field education as a legitimate area of social work inquiry. *Issues in Social Work Education, 19* (1), 2–16.

Noble, C., & Irwin, J. (2009). Social work supervision: An exploration of the current challenges in a rapidly changing social, economic and political environment. *Journal of Social Work, 9,* 345–358.

Parton, N. (1998). Risk, liberalism and child welfare: The need to rediscover uncertainty and ambiguity. *British Journal of Social Work, 28,* 5–27.

Rogers, A. (2001). Nurture, bureaucracy and re-balancing the heart and mind. *Journal of Social Work Practice, 15* (2), 181–191.

Russ, E., Lonne, B., & Darlington, Y. (2009). Using resilience to reconceptualise child protection workforce capacity. *Australian Social Work, 62* (3), 324–338.

Schwartz, R. H., Tiamiyu, M. F., & Dwyer, D. J. (2007). Social worker hope and perceived burnout: The effects of age, years in practice, and setting. *Administration in Social Work, 31* (4), 103–119.

Stalker, C. A., Mandell, D., Frensch, K. M., Harvey, C., & Wright, M. (2007). Child welfare workers who are exhausted yet satisfied with their jobs: How do they do it? *Child & Family Social Work, 12* (2), 182–191.

Townend, M. (2005). Interprofessional supervision from the perspectives of both mental health nurses and other professionals in the field of cognitive behavioural psychotherapy. *Journal of Psychiatric and Mental Health Nursing, 12* (5), 582–588.

Tsui, M. S. (2005). *Social work supervision: Contexts and concepts.* Thousand Oaks, CA: Sage.

Ungar, M. (2004). *Nurturing hidden resilience in troubled youth.* Toronto, Canada: University of Toronto Press.

Ungar, M. (2008). Resilience across cultures. *British Journal of Social Work, 38* (2), 218–235.

van Breda, A. (2011). Resilient workplaces: An initial conceptualization. *Families in Society, 92* (1), 33–40.

External Supervision in Social Work: Power, Space, Risk, and the Search for Safety[1]

Liz Beddoe

School of Counselling, Human Services and Social Work, University of Auckland, Auckland, New Zealand

Abstract

Over the past few decades there has been a trend to separate "clinical" or "professional" supervision of social workers from "line" supervision provided in social services. Professional or clinical supervision is often sourced externally through a private arrangement or contracted out by agencies to individual practitioners of supervision. A number of factors underpin the development of this external supervision including: the perceived imposition of managerial agendas on supervision; the problem of power dynamics within organisations; and a growing "risk" conceptualisation of practitioners' wellbeing. A potential negative impact of this separation of supervision from the "field" of practice is that it privatises supervision in a manner that in itself poses risks. This exploratory paper examines the impact of discourses of risk and safety, space and place within social work supervision and draws links between these aspects. Some material drawn from a small qualitative study of the experiences of six expert supervisors in New Zealand illuminates these themes. A significant finding was that the dominance of compliance and surveillance activities within the public sector was linked to the pursuit of external supervision and that four dominant forms of supervision can be discerned in the current discourse.

Supervision is currently experiencing a resurgence of interest, not in small part due to political and organisational anxiety about risk (Beddoe, 2010; Peach & Horner, 2007) and the recommendations of high profile child abuse inquiries. In the United Kingdom, Lord Laming's review of child protection found that inconsistent provision of supervision remained a persistent problem and recommended improvement (Laming, 2009) Supervision has grown as a practice within the helping professions with diverse models and approaches being developed, each reflecting to large extent the professional habitus of their proponents. There is now a substantial body of literature for each of the professions of counselling, social work, nursing, psychology,

---

[1] Paper accepted under the editorship of Professor Christine Bigby and Dr Jane Maidment.

and psychotherapy (Davys & Beddoe, 2010). There has always been debate about the proper set of functions within the supervisory system and the tensions that exist between these functions within professional and organisational contexts (Payne, 1994). Two features of social work supervision differentiate it from supervision in other professions. The first is that social workers have supervision throughout their career, rather than only while training. The second feature is that supervision has been traditionally practiced "in-house" within organisational settings, hence the strong presence of administrative (Kadushin, 1976) or managerial (Morrison, 2001) functions (Davys & Beddoe, 2010).

Vignette

Jack is a newly-appointed manager of a nongovernmental disability support agency. He is a qualified, registered social worker, with many years experience in the public health system. Jack is surprised to find that all the social workers have external supervision. They have been with the same supervisor for between five and 15 years. When he questions what accountability mechanisms are in place between the agency and the supervisor he meets resistance and is told that all he has to do is approve the invoices for payment. Anything else would be seen as an invasion of privacy.

This story (details changed), told in a supervision training session triggered my interest in the dynamics of "external supervision", some 12 years ago. This paper explores some core issues in contemporary supervision with reference to a recent small study conducted in New Zealand.

Supervision has been a core professional activity in social work since the late 19th century (Tsui & Ho, 1997) and an accepted division of supervisory functions survives. These functions of supervision are commonly labelled administrative, educative, and supportive (Kadushin, 1976). The administrative function describes the participants' accountability to the policies, ethics, and standards that are prescribed by both employing organisations and regulatory bodies. More recent delineations of function are closely aligned to this earlier model. Hughes and Pengelly (1997) acknowledged the growing impact of a risk-averse climate in the "turbulent environment" of social services in the 1990s and identified the foci of supervision as managing service delivery, facilitating practitioners' professional development, and exploration of practitioners' work (Hughes & Pengelly, 1997). Morrison (2001) described four central functions of supervision: competent, accountable performance or practice (managerial); continuing professional development (developmental); personal support (supportive); and engaging the individual with the organisation (mediation function), this latter being a significant addition that originated in a publication by Richards and Payne (1991). The mediative aspect of supervision makes explicit recognition of the complex and competing personal, organisational, and professional agendas present in the supervision encounter (Morrison, 2001).

Bradley, Engelbrecht, and Hojer (2010) further noted that the functions of supervision have remained a relatively stable set of concepts but are not apolitical;

indeed, "in practice they appear less neutral and the time spent proportionately on them is likely to reflect the predominant agenda" (Bradley et al., 2010, p. 777). Bradley et al. (2010) also pointed to an overemphasis on administration, which might reflect an underlying ideology where the agency is management-driven, whereas where supervision has a predominantly supportive focus this is "more likely to promote a person-centred, professional agenda with a different type of power dynamic between worker and supervisor" (Bradley et al., 2010, p. 777). Bradley and Hojer (2009) compared English and Swedish approaches to supervision and noted that in Scandinavian countries a dual approach operates. Supervision provided by external consultants is combined with internal, method-oriented supervision, provided by the line manager of the practitioners (Bradley & Hojer, 2009).

The almost total alignment of supervision and line management in some jurisdictions, and most commonly in statutory (mandated) practice, means that power dynamics are inevitable and need to be addressed (Cousins, 2010). The common depiction of supervision as being both an organisational activity and a professional imperative (Beddoe & Egan, 2009) links to the tensions inherent in social work, where practice is often in state-funded organisations and professional autonomy may be severely limited. These tensions require negotiation of the supervision process and this theme is identified and discussed throughout the literature (Hughes & Pengelly, 1997; Morrison, 2001; Noble & Irwin, 2009; Peach & Horner, 2007). Since the late 1990s there has been an increasing trend in New Zealand toward separation of "clinical" supervision from "line management or administrative supervision" (Cooper, 2006; Morrell, 2001, 2008). This is often referred to as "external supervision", an allusion to the fact that many workers go "outside" their agency for supervision. This development proposes the separation of the organisational accountability for clinical practice from the role of clinical supervisor unless this is specifically contracted between the agency and the external supervisor.

External Supervision: The Debates

External supervision is defined here as supervision that takes place between a practitioner and a supervisor who do not both work for the same employing organisation. The physical space in which this occurs may be different from the worker's normal workplace and it is bounded by complex expectations, which may or may not be covered in a written contract. In the current environment, discourses of risk and vulnerability emanate from anxious, risk-averse governments and impact on supervision. Research suggests the growth of external supervision reflects this broader context (Beddoe, 2010). Discussing risk, Green (2007) stated that "governments and their regulatory agencies are very anxious to control the identification and deployment of risks, given the significance of this process to the allocation of blame" (p. 405).

Supervision can be harnessed to technologies of risk minimisation and, where this appropriation occurs, a shift from a focus on the development of practitioners to the monitoring of their practice occurs (Peach & Horner, 2007). Cooper (2006) argued that managerialist environments encouraged the push towards external supervision and issues of accountability often drive managers to be anxious about supervision. The provision of external supervision can play into the accountability agenda, with supervision rendered a compliance activity to be checked off on the list of mechanisms that aim to ensure safe practice.

Additional arguments in favour of external supervision generally focus on the importance of supervisee choice and direction (Davys, 2005a); supervisory clinical competence (McAuliffe & Sudbery, 2005); unhealthy organisational culture (Hawkins & Shohet, 2006); concern about surveillance (Peach & Horner, 2007); and concerns about power differentials in the supervisory relationship when it is a dual relationship (e.g., the supervisor is a line manager) (Gilbert, 2001; McAuliffe & Sudbery, 2005). Supervisee choice was important, especially in relation to group membership and professional identity, as reported by Davys (2005a), where participant choice was a major indicator of satisfaction. Consideration of supervisee and supervisor characteristics particularly in relation to ethnicity, culture, gender, age, and professional and theoretical orientation are also considered to be important (Davys, 2005b; Hair & O'Donoghue, 2009; Tsui & Ho, 1997).

Organisational Culture and Surveillance

Cooper (2006) noted that supervision was a "highly individualised practice" (p. 29), often valued for the privacy of a one-to-one relationship, with meetings held behind closed doors. Confidentiality is highly valued by practitioners, and one significant factor that differentiates external supervision from a line management approach to supervision is the expectation that an external supervisor will hold less information about the practitioner, including administrative, educational, career, and personal issues, which may be well known by an internal supervisor. Cooper's research on supervision within a large mental health service (Cooper, 2006; Cooper & Anglem, 2003) found that there was "a degree of mistrust between practitioners and line managers, as line managers have comprehensive administrative information about practitioners, and this may lower levels of confidentiality" (Cooper, 2006, p. 29). Where supervision is a private arrangement between practitioners, conducted "outside the managerial gaze, confidentiality will have a high priority" (Cooper, 2006, p. 29). Difficulties of access to *social work* supervision within organisations are also common (McAuliffe & Sudbery, 2005). Power and aspects of organisational culture that stifle critical reflection may drive the use of external supervision, and McAuliffe and Sudbery (2005) found that research participants with external supervisors were more likely to have raised ethical dilemmas in supervision having requested "dedicated time for clarification of ethical dimensions and problem-solving" (p. 28). These researchers noted that some workers reported a critical position on internal supervision where it is linked to control and managerial concerns (McAuliffe & Sudbery, 2005).

Supervision is generally accepted as a core process within social work, despite these unsettling influences that stem from the new public management (Jones, 2004) and other upheavals faced during recent times of turbulence (Noble & Irwin, 2009). While the literature predominantly portrays supervision as facilitative and supportive, interpretations of government policy promote supervision as risk focussed and a vaccine against mistakes (Beddoe, 2010). The critique of supervision as a form of surveillance is not new; although it has been notably stronger in nursing, as noted in Johns' concern that "supervision...becomes an opportunity to shape the practitioner into organisationally preferred ways of practice, even whilst veiled as being in the practitioner's best interests" (Johns, 2001, p. 140). Gilbert (2001) suggested that as supervision can "demonstrate the subtle but pervasive exercise of power that operates to maintain a level of surveillance upon the activity of professionals" (p. 200). For supervisors, the focus on scrutiny of practice decisions can become a constant source of stress as is worker safety. Supervision becomes a central plank in a professional safety discourse, as O'Donoghue, Munford, and Trlin (2006) found where:

> supervision was also depicted as an accountability forum... as well as "shared responsibility for decisions". Safety was concerned with: the respondent's safety, client and supervisee safety, enabling "safe practice" and the provision of a "safety net" for the worker. (p. 83)

Anxiety abounds about adverse practice outcomes, which may range from simple errors that moderately threaten reputation; negative comment on the organisation; fear of serious harm to service users, patients, staff, or the public; and the publicity attached to these adverse events (Kemshall, 2010). When anxiety overwhelms other more positive approaches to practice, innovation may become too risky (Beddoe, 2009). Supervisors reported that reliance on risk-assessment tools rather than reflection promoted more reactive and mechanistic practice creativity may be reduced (Beddoe, 2010). Gillingham's research in Australia has indicated that checklists in supervision may reduce some of the anxiety that supervisors feel but not necessarily improve the practice (Gillingham, 2006; Gillingham & Bromfield, 2008). In a similar vein, Stanley argued that "the paradox of risk is that a surface approach and application to it actually increases risks to children, those with mental illness and others of vulnerability" (Stanley, 2010, p. 38).

Space, Place, and Power

My previous research (Beddoe, 2009) has explored the layers of discourse in professional practice in organisational settings. Supervision is a highly specific form of professional communication and discourse and is thus both influenced by and has influence on the spaces and places in which it is enacted and spoken. Bernstein's concepts of "vertical" and "horizontal" discourse are useful to consider here when considering what kinds of practice might be reflected in and by supervision in social work. Bernstein (1999) suggested that academic (in this case, theory informed and systematic supervision) and "everyday" knowledge (here, perhaps the more person-centred narrative traditions of supervision) represent different, incompatible knowledge forms that cannot be successfully integrated. Vertical discourse takes the form of a coherent, explicit, and systematically principled structure, hierarchically organised (in the sciences), or "a series of specialised languages with specialised modes of interrogations and specialised criteria for the production and circulation of texts, as in the social sciences and humanities" (Bernstein, 1999, p. 159). Williams and Wilson (2010) explained that "access to vertical discourse is controlled by strong 'distributive rules' which regulate power relations between social groups by distributing to them different forms of knowledge, 'consciousness' and identity" (p. 422). Thus, line management supervision might be characterised by rules, risk assessment checklists, in the realm of compliant bureaucracy. Such hierarchical supervision relationships may render culture and difference invisible, or contain racist or homophobic dynamics and become oppressive (Hair & O'Donoghue, 2009; Hernandez & McDowell, 2010).

By contrast, horizontal discourses are the "common sense" kinds of knowledge available to those who share understandings within in a community and activated in everyday social practice. Bernstein (1999) described horizontal discourses as "likely to be oral, local, context dependent and specific, tacit, multi-layered, and contradictory across but not within contexts" (p. 159). Horizontal discourses are informally acquired, either tacitly, by behaviours observed or modelled in face-to-face encounters in relationships in social contexts. Supervision in which power inequalities and barriers to free expression are minimised might fit this latter form of discourse, and thus be more grounded in the reflective but structured conversations suggested in reflective learning supervision (Davys & Beddoe, 2010) or in structured critical reflection (Fook & Gardner, 2007). Supervision that is cognisant of the cultural and socioeconomic oppression of non dominant groups, whether as social workers or service-users, is needed if supervision "can successfully encourage cultural relevancy and the pursuit of social justice" (Hair & O'Donoghue, 2009, p. 70). Oppressive dynamics are not inevitable, but without addressing these tensions supervision may reflect wider organisational and societal oppressive dynamics, and this is a powerful driver of external "cultural supervision" in New Zealand (Davys, 2005b).

Is the physical place in which these reflective encounters take place equally as important as the more mutable "space" in which identity and power factors play? Both notions of space and place frequently occur as terms used in the discussion of supervision. Busse (2009) suggested that supervision has become somewhat detached from its core of reflective practice and has

> become frayed at the edges as a result of its almost uncurbed expansion in a horizontal direction (its development from an individual setting to being located at the edge of organisational consultancy) and in a vertical direction (into professional fields other than social work, including profit areas). (p. 165)

Supervision has also become detached from the tradition of individuals meeting in their shared workplace. It is this removal to an external space that O'Donoghue et al. (2006) described where practitioners were concerned with:

> The *location* where supervision occurred, its availability, the type of *space* provided by supervision and the *place* that supervision was for them. For the respondents an external location, (i.e. *outside of the agency*) . . . conducted in a relaxed atmosphere, within a *space provided* for offloading, discussion, and reflection, were key features. (Italics added) (p. 84)

The "place" can be significant as a safety-zone, away from the busy workplace, removed from the tensions inherent in crisis work: "The respondents described [supervision] as the *place* where they connected with their supervisor, profession, peer and group; shared their frustrations and successes; could be challenged; and could learn and develop" [Italics added], (O'Donoghue et al., 2006, p. 84).

For Busse (2009) the location of external supervision away from the office is an attempt to achieve a more reflective, democratic space:

> Supervision, as has become clearer, is an exclusive *space* for the reflexive achievement of *distance* from working life, but it is not a *space* that can be kept free of the logic of the latter, or one from which this reality can be locked out. [Italics added] (p. 162)

The place can also be problematic. "The shortcomings [of external supervision] are that it is too removed from practice, isolated from the organisation and *takes place in secluded rooms*" [Italics added], (Bradley et al., 2010, p. 784–785).

Issues of power and control are at the heart of these discomforts and power is the most problematic aspect of line management supervision. Supervision relationships cannot be easily sheltered from the operation of policy in action. Gilbert and Powell (2010) noted that "power relations operating via the most mundane interactions between managers, social workers, service users and carers enable the formation and shifting of alliances between political and non-political authorities" (p. 12).

So, if the space and place in which supervision is conducted is fraught with difficulties and power is the main factor is external supervision the answer? It is assumed that external supervision lessens the impact of power and authority issues. Supervisees will thus have greater freedom to express themselves and presumably to ventilate about organisational issues. There are a number of pitfalls in the separation of supervision from clinical accountability. There may be an ambiguous mandate for dealing with issues of poor performance where supervisors become aware of performance matters but have no mandate or clear contract to address these. There is the potential for unhealthy collusion where there are grievances in the practitioner relationships with line managers and the separation of supervision from practice may deepen the experience of the gulf between "management" and "practice" and thus reduce the flow of information between the layers of the organisation.

Method

Conversations with "External" Supervisors about Risk and Safety in Supervision

In order to explore the impact of the risk-averse environment on supervision, experienced supervisors were invited to participate in an exploration of supervision in the risk society (as reported in Beddoe, 2010). The broad themes arising in the main study were: (a) if allowed, risk obsession stifles professional growth opportunities in supervision; (b) good supervision is determined more by process not content; (c) balancing the functions of supervision is required and lastly; and (d) separation of managerial and professional aspects of supervision is ideal, with an unanticipated subtheme emerging concerning risk and the management of external supervision relationships (Beddoe, 2010).

Participants

Six experienced supervisors were invited to participate in the study. Interviews were designed to shed light on the challenges of supervision practice in the current climate. All six participants had considerable involvement and interest in supervision in the social services in New Zealand. Participants were selected for the research according to the following criteria: they were qualified social workers; held supervision qualifications, or had undertaken teaching, practice development, or research in the field; had supervised staff in more than one field of practice, and at least five years supervision experience. Given the small number of participants and the purposive selection, these experiences cannot be viewed as representative of New Zealand supervisors. The participants had from seven to 20 years supervision experience and all had supervised both within their employment in social service organisations and as external supervisors.

Themes

The broad themes for exploration were: supervision and line management; influences of recent regulation of social work in New Zealand; supervisory focus on the key traditional functions of supervision and organisational compliance pressures; any strain experienced between person-centred, facilitative supervision and managerial or compliance activities; and awareness of the current discussion of surveillance of professionals within in the risk society (Beddoe, 2010). That a focus on external supervision emerged in the interview data was spontaneous but not unexpected.

Results

Compliance, Surveillance, and Supervision

The dominance of compliance and surveillance activities within public sector regimes of audit and quality management was a common point of reference for participants in the study, as a reason for external supervision. Lucy[1] noted that "my concern is

---

[1] Pseudonyms are used throughout the paper to protect the privacy of the individuals concerned.

that what's actually happening is that . . . supervision becomes tick box compliance". Lucy felt the focus on compliance altered the focus of supervision:

> There is not sufficient high level understanding about the reflective nature [of supervision] so all that we're doing is actually if you like reinforcing, will end up being [what Proctor calls] normative supervision which may also be about risk management. (Lucy)

Risk management reflected managerial concerns: "Risk management is actually management supervision. I don't think it's the same as reflective supervision . . . let's not confuse [management supervision] with whatever you want to call it, professional, clinical, reflective supervision" (Lucy); and "When I think about it, that's also what the problem in child protection is probably. They turn up at supervision . . . with their list of case load" (Mary).

Participants wanted supervision to avoid an overemphasis on compliance; and it was also important that external supervision did not go in that direction, given the dominance of compliance inside organisations: "The line management stuff and the surveillance stuff needs to be internal rather than external and if you push external supervision to be like that then you lose that space for reflection" (Andrea).

> I think even though my social workers are really comfortable in supervision there is always that aspect of feeling under scrutiny that can make it a little bit more of a nervous exercise and where you probably do call on the compliance...you have people who turn up but they're actually in a resistance frame so you don't have particularly good quality supervision, you have all the undercurrents. (Angie)

Angie felt that power often underpinned the discomfort with line management supervision and the move towards external supervision. As a professional leader she was conscious that social workers want to keep management and reflective supervision separate: "There is again always that slightly unnamed aspect of power. When people start resisting or actually feeling not particularly comfortable in your agency, the next thing you can guarantee is they'll ask for external [supervision]" (Angie).

Thus, quality of supervision was also a significant issue in internal supervision and participants noted that that it is really hard to get that balance when in a workplace.

> Crikey, I think I might have made a really big challenge you know creating that no blame culture whilst also having a culture of scrutiny about practice. [It is] difficult, something that I haven't managed to achieve and I'm really keen to achieve it. You know it's a safe environment for people to discover their learning edge. (Rose)

Emotional Safety: Social Workers at Risk

One of the major arguments for external supervision is that it provides an opportunity to offer emotional support that is untainted by power relations and issues of confidentiality. Thus, the external supervisor becomes seen as an advocate for stressed and troubled workers. Stanford (2010) noted that "the rhetoric of risk, however, also extends to social workers who are constructed as 'at risk' from clients (increasingly considered to pose a physical and/or emotional/psychological threat), critical colleagues and managers . . . and they are 'a risk' to vulnerable clients if they do not identify and respond appropriately to apparent risk" (p. 1067). Angie commented on the additional risk where a supervisor was stressed:

> I think one of the most dangerous things I've seen is supervisors who are actually really anxious and so the worker, often because social workers are generally quite empathetic, picks up that their supervisor is not in a good head space and they shield them and [then we see] behaviours coming out, that start to tell you that the worker is trying to contain too much. (Angie)

Knowing when practitioners are "at risk" or "a risk", to employ Stanford's (2010) depictions, emerged as one of the concerns for external supervisors. All participants noted a tendency to rely on reported performance rather than the full 360° information collected through day-to-day interaction and observation of practitioner performance in teams, case consultations, meetings, and internal supervision. Issues of duty of care to practitioners and service users can remain unclear and yet may be vitally significant when things go wrong. For these reasons, Rose, who had provided internal and external supervision, felt that she was quite unusual in her view that supervision and line management were perhaps better undertaken by the same person:

> My experience of people being engaged in external supervision is that they rely entirely on report from the supervisor. People can be in a quite a difficult work environment, you know either performing not so well or things can be going on that [need to be] attended to but my experience is that they're not so often addressed in external supervision. (Rose)

There is potential for an unhealthy triangulation of practitioner, line manager, and clinical supervisor and so sufficient attention must be paid to the clarity of the mandate for supervision and lines of communication (Davys & Beddoe, 2010). Contracts are important and a line manager may be relieved of responsibility to ensure all aspects of the monitoring of personal and practice safety issues in the workplace:

> I think the other risk [is where] a supervisee is defined as being at risk in terms of their behaviour or their health or something and an external supervisor doesn't know. That's the bit that I think is dangerous for the supervisor because you don't know what . . . the supervisee chooses not to tell you for whatever reason. (Lucy)

Managing accountability in external supervision was often linked to concerns about supervisor accountability:

> You don't always know whether there's honesty happening between the supervisee and the organisation so yeah it is a risk you have to manage... I do think about it... particularly where a supervisee has said to their managers that yes they've taken [an

issue] to supervision and then you wonder...what sort of expectation of me does the organisation have? (Andrea)

Andrea's method for dealing with these concerns was to develop a strong tripartite contract with the supervisee, the organisation, and herself. Thus, external supervision requires diligent attention to relationships and at times this may require more input than busy managers might want, as Andrea stated: "often it's hard to get all the parties together to talk, you have conversations on the phone, there's that feeling of the confidentiality lying between the supervisee and supervisor". Andrea and others also noted that the financial arrangement challenged expectations of confidentiality: "And how much is the organisation required to know because they're paying for it?" (Andrea).

There was a sense that private supervisors must be willing to accept the heavy burden of clinical accountability, which could become a major issue with regulation and thus greater investigation and potential litigation of complaints. All participants felt that contracts and at least annual meetings were essential to manage the risks, confirming the best practice suggested by Morrell (2001, 2008) and Davys (2007).

Supervisors noted the importance of their own choices in offering supervision. Putting limits on numbers and restricting their scope or focus of practice enabled them to put some boundaries up for their own safety and accountability. For Margaret, one way to limit her "risk" was to be clear about who she would agree to supervise:

> I was thinking today about who I'm supervising and who I choose not to take because of that surveillance piece so I don't feel compromised in the context of my private practice. Does that make sense? I don't for instance supervise [statutory] social workers because I don't have the knowledge. (Margaret)

Mary could see the value of both internal and external supervision:

> In the past, I've tended to think that in an ideal world it is more cost effective ... if the line manager (if the relationship...and the conditions are right in the organisation) could provide the so-called clinical supervision. That doesn't happen very often but I guess I think back to some of my supervision from a line manager and thought that we integrated it quite well. (Mary)

Discussion

It is suggested that there are four dominant forms of supervision: internal managerial, internal reflective, external professional, and external personal, as shown in Figures 1 and 2.

Rather than see internal and external supervision as polar opposites, it is useful to see a continuum of forms with different foci and attempt to capture the best features. At one end of this continuum, *internal managerial* supervision takes place inside the organisation and is mostly focused on task and process. At the other end, *external personal supervision* is worker-focused and centres mainly on the narrative brought

| Internal —External: Process, Focus, and Aims → |

Internal Managerial	Internal Reflective	External Professional	External Personal
• Process based • Organisation centred • Systems focus • Technologies of practice • Task compliance	• Knowledge based • Worker/user focused • Reflective practice • Development	• Knowledge based • Worker/user focused • Professional identity • Critical Reflection	• Narrative based • Worker focused • Use-of self focus • Emotional damage control

Figure 1 The processes, foci, and aims of the four dominant forms of supervision: internal managerial, internal reflective, external professional, and external personal.

into the supervision space by the worker (Figure 1). To return to Jack's story from the introduction, this is the exclusive arrangement found by him in his new job. This type of supervision will highly value the space for worker ventilation of feelings, thus echoing O'Donoghue et al.'s (2006) findings about the need for a safe place to connect and reflect on use-of-self. The study participants all recognised that within a strong commitment to supervision, both internal and external supervision could be reflective. All valued the promotion of reflective practice as an integral part of supervision, which should be separated from the technologies of accountability and compliance. In advocating this approach they did not suggest that compliance was not important; rather that it should be largely removed from the private reflective space of supervision.

These participants' views have confirmed that tensions between managerial accountability and professional autonomy remain an ever-present issue in social work supervision. The ability to hold these tensions within a trusting relationship with practitioners is an essential competency for managers and supervisors alike. The alternative seems to be the total removal of the reflective supervision effort to the private sector, leaving internal supervision in statutory agencies too often at the mercy of dominating managerial concerns. Cooper's (2006) research noted the tendency for practitioners within one organisation to regard supervision as a

> predominantly private arrangement between two individuals to ensure the highest possible quality of care and professional standards … This arrangement, driven by the supervisees, is evidenced in particular by supervisees choosing the most appropriate supervisors for their needs, sometimes from another profession, entering into mostly verbal contracts. (p. 29)

Furthermore, and significantly, Cooper (2006) noted "the general feeling that they do not need to give line managers any feedback about supervision" (p. 29). It needs to be asked whether as a profession social work is willing to put at risk one of the anchors of our profession. Indeed, that was Jack's concern when he told the story on a supervision course. How did he know whether the supervision was supporting safe practice? The expert supervisors in this current study suggest that the practice of supervision is evolving as awareness of multiple and complex accountabilities create some new ideas about supervision. Importantly, they did not exclude the possibility that internal supervision could meet needs. Their emphasis was on relationship and transparency.

Do We Really Want to Leave it to Market Forces?

External supervision, located as it is outside of the agency, may well allow more intensive focus on clinical issues and personal professional development rather than organisational concerns. Figure 2 delineates aspects of the four forms of supervision with reference to professional inquiry, emotion, and risk identity. External supervision may provide a place in which knowledge can be utilised and created, although the participants in this study were not specifically asked about knowledge use. While there was little discussion of use of knowledge in supervision, there was a strong identification of supervision with professional identity and competence. In addition, this external supervision arrangement may increase the likelihood that supervision actually does take place. In busy agency settings, supervision can often be neglected or deferred to accommodate the latest crisis unless it is made a high priority by management. Jack's predecessor had liked this arrangement as he could tick supervision off as covered.

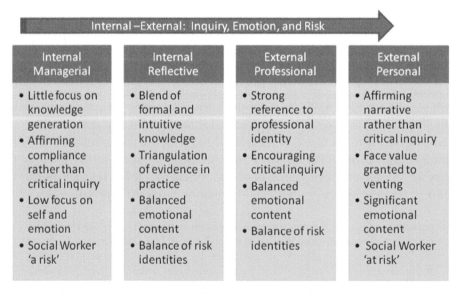

Figure 2 The inquiry, emotions, and risk elements of the four dominant forms of supervision: internal managerial, internal reflective, external professional, and external personal.

However, as Busse (2009) has pointed out, the widespread development of external supervision has effectively privatised it. Supervision has to some extent left the traditional site within the public or non governmental organisation into the private sector where it has a market value. A further weakness of shifting supervision to this "arm's length" position is that it may diminish professional efficacy to exert pressure for organisational change (Bradley et al., 2010), as supervisors' ability to mediate between frontline workers and management (Morrison, 2001) is diminished by their external status. As a private commodity, purchased sometimes by the individual practitioner, more often by their agency, it becomes less visible, less a collective good linked to shared professional aspirations. This trend may be seen as both a consequence and a reflection of the adoption of the "market" model in social services. It reflects the "purchaser-provider" split so favoured by "new right" economic arguments. In the ultimate market model, supervision is a commodity to be purchased, as part of the cost of "human resources" for the enterprise. If "employee assistance" and "health and safety" can all be purchased in the market place at lower cost to the organisation, why not supervision? Figure 2 illustrates the impact of this privatisation of supervision. The diagram suggests that on a continuum of "internal managerial" to "external personal" the focus reflects Stanford's (2010) "risk identities". In the "internal" space, the focus may settle on the practitioner as "a risk", while an "external personal" model places the social worker "at risk" in a private space where venting is encouraged and the supervisee's feelings are held with minimal challenge. Jack was very concerned that a worker who was displaying signs of burnout and disillusionment was unwilling to discuss this at all, even when her behaviour was causing stress in the team. Her emotional wellbeing in the work was not an area she wished to discuss and Jack's attempt to arrange a meeting with her external supervisor present for support was unwelcome.

Conclusions

The author's view is that supervision is a complex, multifaceted process, which occupies contested space between the employing organisation and the employed professional social worker. It is supervision that is at the core of practice for service-based professionals, where a sense of shared responsibility for the effectiveness and safety of the practice is essential. If we separate the functions of this complex process from each other, what mechanisms can exist in order to ensure that the safety of all of the participants (practitioner, service delivery manager, clinical supervisor, clients and other service users, and indeed the profession itself) in the supervisory process? In an increasingly litigious world, how do we define and manage the duty of care that exists between the parties? Does the absence of legitimated authority in the supervisor lead to a lack of real challenge? What can supervisors do to check out other perspectives?

Several areas for further exploration are signalled in this paper. The first relates to the supervision discourse. We know so little about what in reality happens in supervision; for example, how much formal knowledge is discussed or interrogated and the extent to which critical reflection is promoted, although it is a common assumption that external supervision will better support reflective practice. A second issue concerns education and standards for supervision. In New Zealand, Australia, and many other countries, supervisor education is not required and yet supervision is often mandated (Social Workers Registration Board, 2009). O'Donoghue (2010) has made strong recommendations for the development of supervisor education and evaluation, and, given mandatory supervision requirements, further research by professional bodies is needed.

The participants in this study strongly support what Noble and Irwin (2009) termed "the joint and equal...experience" (p. 355) of how to democratise the supervision process so as to move it towards a more equal and socially aware experience. While external supervision may provide some answers on the surface, in reality even those who provide it pose serious questions about safety, transparency, and the wellbeing of the profession.

References

Beddoe, L. (2009). Creating continuous conversation: Social workers and learning organizations. *Social Work Education-The International Journal, 28*, 722–736.

Beddoe, L. (2010). Surveillance or reflection: Professional supervision in "the risk society". *British Journal of Social Work, 40*, 1279–1296.

Beddoe, L., & Egan, R. (2009). Social work supervision. In M. Connolly & L. Harms (Eds.), *Social work: Contexts and practice* (2nd ed, pp. 410–422). Melbourne: Oxford University Press.

Bernstein, B. (1999). Vertical and horizontal discourse: An essay. *British Journal of Sociology of Education, 20*, 157–173.

Bradley, G., & Hojer, S. (2009). Supervision reviewed: Reflections on two different social work models in England and Sweden. *European Journal of Social Work, 12*, 71–85.

Bradley, G., Engelbrecht, L., & Hojer, S. (2010). Supervision: A force for change? Three stories told. *International Social Work, 53*, 773–790.

Busse, S. (2009). Supervision between critical reflection and practical action. *Journal of Social Work Practice, 23*, 159–173.

Cooper, L. (2006). Clinical supervision: Private arrangement or managed process? *Social Work Review, 18*, 21–30.

Cooper, L., & Anglem, J. (2003). *Clinical supervision in mental health.* Adelaide: Australian Centre for Community Services Research, Flinders University and Anglicare SA.

Cousins, C. (2010). "Treat me don't beat me": Exploring supervisory games and their effect on poor performance management. *Practice: Social Work in Action, 22*, 281–292.

Davys, A. (2005a). Supervision: Is what we want what we need? Weaving together the strands of supervision. In L. Beddoe, J. Worrall, & F. Howard (Eds.),, 2004, *Conference Proceedings* (pp. 15–24), Auckland: University of Auckland.

Davys, A. (2005b). At the heart of the matter: Culture as a function of supervision. *Social Work Review, 17*, 3–12.

Davys, A. (2007). Active participation in supervision: A supervisee's guide. In D. Wepa (Ed.), *Clinical supervision in Aotearoa/New Zealand: A health perspective* (pp. 26–42). Auckland: Pearson Education.

Davys, A., & Beddoe, L. (2010). *Best practice in supervision: A guide for the helping professions.* London: Jessica Kingsley.

Fook, J., & Gardner, F. (2007). *Practising critical reflection: A resource handbook.* Maidenhead: Open University Press.

Gilbert, T. (2001). Reflective practice and clinical supervision: Meticulous rituals of the confessional. *Journal of Advanced Nursing, 36,* 199–205.

Gilbert, T., & Powell, J. L. (2010). Power and social work in the United Kingdom: A Foucauldian excursion. *Journal of Social Work, 10,* 3–22.

Gillingham, P. (2006). Risk assessment in child protection: Problem rather than solution. *Australian Social Work, 59,* 86–98.

Gillingham, P., & Bromfield, L. (2008). Child protection, risk assessment and blame ideology. *Children Australia, 33,* 18–24.

Green, D. (2007). Risk and social work practice. *Australian Social Work, 60,* 395–409.

Hair, H. J., & O'Donoghue, K. (2009). Culturally relevant, socially just social work supervision: Becoming visible through a social constructionist lens. *Journal of Ethnic and Cultural Diversity in Social Work, 18,* 70–88.

Hawkins, P., & Shohef, R. (2006). *Supervision in the helping professions* (3rd ed.). Maidenhead: Open University Press.

Hernández, P., & McDowell, T. (2010). Intersectionality, power, and relational safety in context: Key concepts in clinical supervision. *Training and Education in Professional Psychology, 4,* 29–35.

Hughes, L., & Pengelly, P. (1997). *Staff supervision in a turbulent environment: Managing process and task in front-line services.* London: Jessica Kingsley.

Johns, C. (2001). Depending on the intent and emphasis of the supervisor, clinical supervision can be a different experience. *Journal of Nursing Management, 9,* 139–145.

Jones, M. (2004). Supervision, learning and transformative practices. In N. Gould & M. Baldwin (Eds.), *Social work, critical reflection and the learning organisation* (pp. 11–22). Aldershot: Ashgate.

Kadushin, A. (1976). *Supervision in social work.* New York, NY: Columbia University Press.

Laming, The Lord, (2009). *The protection of children in England: A progress report.* London: HM Government. The Stationery Office.

Kemshall, H. (2010). Risk rationalities in contemporary social work policy and practice. *British Journal of Social Work, 40,* 1247–1262.

McAuliffe, D., & Sudbery, J. (2005). "Who do I tell?" Support and consultation in cases of ethical conflict. *Journal of Social Work, 5,* 21–43.

Morrell, M. (2001). External supervision-confidential or accountable? An exploration of the relationship between agency, supervisor and supervisee. *Social Work Review, 13,* 36–41.

Morrell, M. (2008). Supervision contracts revisited: Towards a negotiated agreement. *Social Work Review, 20,* 22–31.

Morrison, T. (2001). *Staff supervision in social care: Making a real difference for staff and service users.* Brighton: Pavilion.

Noble, C., & Irwin, J. (2009). Social work supervision: An exploration of the current challenges in a rapidly changing social, economic and political environment. *Journal of Social Work, 9,* 345–358.

O'Donoghue, K. (2010). *Towards the construction of social work supervision in Aotearoa New Zealand: A study of the perspectives of social work practitioners and supervisors.* Unpublished doctoral thesis: Massey University, Palmerston North, New Zealand.

O'Donoghue, K., Munford, R., & Trlin, A. (2006). What's best about social work supervision according to Association members. *Social Work Review, 18,* 79–92.

Payne, M. (1994). Personal supervision in social work. In A. Connor & S. E. Black (Eds.), *Performance review and quality in social care* (pp. 43–58). London: Jessica Kingsley.

Peach, J., & Horner, N. (2007). Using supervision: Support or surveillance. In M. Lymbery & K. Postle (Eds.), *Social work: A companion to learning* (pp. 228–239). London: Sage.

Richards, M., & Payne, C. (1991). *Staff supervision in child protection work.* London: National Institute for Social Work.

Social Workers Registration Board, S. (2009). *Supervision expectations for registered social workers: Policy statement.* Wellington, NZ: SWRB. Retrieved April 1, 2011, from http://www.swrb.org.nz/files/Policies/RegSupervisionExpectationsRegSW.pdf.

Stanford, S. (2010). Speaking back" to fear: Responding to the moral dilemmas of risk in social work practice. *British Journal of Social Work, 40,* 1065–1080.

Stanley, T. (2010). Working with "risk": It's more than just an assessment idea. *Aotearoa New Zealand Social Work Review, 22,* 37–43.

Tsui, M. S., & Ho, W. S. (1997). In search of a comprehensive model of social work supervision. *Clinical Supervisor, 16,* 181–205.

Williams, C., & Wilson, S. (2010). Pedagogies for social justice: Did Bernstein get it wrong? *International Journal of Inclusive Education, 14,* 417–434.

Professional Supervision: A Workforce Retention Strategy for Social Work?

Phoebe Chiller & Beth R. Crisp

School of Health and Social Development, Deakin University, Geelong, Victoria, Australia

Abstract

Retaining social workers in the workforce is a significant challenge and a considerable amount of research has focused on identifying and examining the reasons why social workers choose to leave the profession. This paper presents findings collected as part of a small-scale exploratory study into why some social workers have chosen to remain in the social work profession for many years and who consider themselves to be passionate about their careers. In particular, the paper focuses on the potential of effective professional supervision as a factor that can facilitate social worker workforce retention. Supervision was mentioned by all participants in the study as being important for their wellbeing, either throughout their social work career or at particular points along the way, and supervision was also cited as one of the reasons they were still social workers. On the basis of this research, the authors argue that regular professional supervision can increase the retention rate of social worker employees; and it is, therefore, false economy not to allocate sufficient resources for effective supervision.

Social work is both a rewarding and a stressful occupation. Every day social workers tackle the issues that many of the general public prefer to ignore. Furthermore, social workers are often required to work with individuals who do not wish to be helped and who can be aggressive or even violent towards them (Coffey, Dudgill, & Tattersall, 2009). This ongoing exposure to trauma and hardship can make social work an emotionally draining and demanding profession (e.g., Dollard, Winefield, & Winefield, 2001; Guy, Newman, & Mastacci, 2008; Russ, Lonne, & Darlington, 2009). Added to this, many social workers have reported a lack of feedback or reward for their efforts, unless they are being blamed for their actions (Guy et al., 2008; Pines, 1993).

Social workers also must practice in what is currently, at least in Australia, a very testing political climate. Many social work organisations are also chronically under-resourced and economic rationalism can result in social work organisations being forced to strive for efficiency rather than effectiveness. This means that many social workers are experiencing very high caseloads and are expected to do more with increasingly fewer resources. They are also expected to work more quickly (Brewer & Shapard, 2004; Halbesleben, 2008), and often with little formal support, supervision, or guidance (Dollard et al., 2001). This pressure can translate into a negative organisational culture, poor staff morale, and the breakdown of peer networks (Morazes, Benton, Clark, & Jacquet, 2010; Russ et al., 2009), and it has been suggested that it is these organisational factors, rather than work with clients, that in fact creates the most negative stress for social workers (Dollard et al., 2001).

This culmination of stressors has been linked to the high prevalence of burnout among social workers (e.g., Brewer & Shapard, 2004; Guy et al., 2008; Pines, 1993; Schaufeli, Maslach, & Marek, 1993), which in turn is often linked to the poor retention rates and high turnover of staff that is strongly evident in the social work field (e.g., Curtis, Moriarty, & Netten, 2010; Halbesleben, 2008; Russ et al., 2009; Saakvitne & Pearlman, 1996) and a key contributor to shortages of social workers. Many social workers leave the field prematurely, with their average expected working life being notably shorter than that of similar professionals. A recent British study suggested that the average working life for a social worker was 8 years, compared to 15 years for nurses, 25 years for doctors, and 28 years for pharmacists (Curtis et al., 2010). It has also been found that newly qualified social workers in several countries, including Australia, Sweden, and the UK (Healy, Meagher, & Cullin, 2009) and Ireland (Burns, 2011), are disproportionately employed in highly stressful positions, such as child protection, which many social workers aim to leave as soon as possible, and some of whom leave social work altogether. Among those that do stay in the profession, staff turnover is high, meaning that few social workers stay in the same job for any great length of time (Curtis et al., 2010; Russ et al., 2009). Even fewer stay in direct practice, with movement to other areas such as management being common (Healy et al., 2009). Poor retention rates and high staff turnover means that organisations must expend already scarce resources on constantly recruiting and training new staff (Dollard et al., 2001); and the consistency, quality, and effectiveness of services provided to clients is also left markedly reduced (Brewer & Shapard, 2004; Russ et al., 2009).

Although much is known about why a great number of social workers do not stay in the profession, much less is known about why others do stay and continue to work in highly stressful conditions for many years (Burns, 2011). There have been several recommendations aimed at encouraging retention. Foremost among these has been the call to recognise the importance of regular and supportive supervision (e.g., Brewer & Shapard, 2004; Kickul & Posig, 2001; Stalker, Mandell, Frensch, Harvey, & Wright, 2007). Associated with this have been calls for transparent management styles that encourage open communication (Dollard et al., 2001; Halbesleben, 2008), along with opportunities for ongoing training and professional development (Healy et al.,

2009; Kanter, 2007). Some writers have emphasised the importance of a supportive organisational culture and morale that allows managers and workers to "look out for" each other (Guy et al., 2008; Morrison, 2007). In addition to developing good relationships between managers and their staff, good peer relationships with other social workers are also posited as facilitating the retention of social workers (Anderson, 2000; Morazes et al., 2010; Pines & Kafry, 2001). Hence, peer debriefing strategies and peer support programs are an integral part of some workplaces (Halbesleben, 2008; Russ et al., 2009; Saakvitne & Pearlman, 1996).

This paper considers the role of supervision in contributing to workforce retention in social work. The data were collected as part of an exploratory study seeking to understand what factors contribute to social workers not only remaining in direct practice in the long term, but continuing to be passionate about their work. Professional supervision has long been regarded as having three distinct functions that involve management, support, and professional development, and typically involving a less experienced supervisee and more experienced supervisor, who meet to discuss the work of the former (Davys & Beddoe, 2010). However, it has also been recognised that the experience and expectations of individual social workers do not always incorporate all of these functions (Crisp & Cooper, 1998), that supervisory arrangements can be more ad hoc than planned, and that supervision can often be provided by those considered to be peers (Green Lister & Crisp, 2005). Hence, it is the participants' understandings of supervision that have been presented in this paper, rather than those of the authors.

Method

Participants

In line with the aims of the study, participants needed to possess a minimum of 10 years of experience as a social worker, be employed in a position that included a direct practice role, and have identified themselves as passionate about their job. A brochure outlining the aims of the study was emailed to 10 experienced social workers who were associated with the social work program at Deakin University. Recipients of the email were asked to consider volunteering for the study if they met the participant criteria and to forward the email on to any other social workers they knew, who might be eligible to participate.

Six social workers from across the State of Victoria volunteered for the study. They were aged between their thirties to fifties and 5 were female. The number of years they had worked as a social worker ranged from 10 to 30 years. At the time of interview, 4 participants were employed in the health sector and 2 in the community service sector. However, all had worked in a range of positions during their career with several reporting periods of employment in positions widely regarded within the profession as being among the most stressful due to the nature of the work or the organisational context in which practice occurred. Summary information for each participant is presented in Table 1.

Table 1 Participants: Current Employment and Number of Years Working as a Social Worker

Name[1]	Current employment sector	Number of years as social worker
Alison	Health	18
Cathy	Health	10
Dianne	Health	25
Fiona	Health	22
Kate	Community services	18
Thomas	Community services	30

[1]Pseudonyms have been used throughout this paper to preserve the anonymity of participants.

Data Collection

Potential participants contacted the first author to arrange a time for interview. At this time, a plain language statement outlining the nature of the study was sent to them in accordance with the approval for the study from the Deakin University Human Ethics Advisory Group.

Semistructured interviews were conducted by the first author. Interview questions required participants to reflect on their social work career and why they considered they had remained within the profession when many others had not. In particular, they were asked about their passion for social work, strategies they had adopted to deal with the stresses of their position, and what advice they would offer to a new graduate commencing a career in social work. Interviews ranged from 20 minutes to 1 hour in duration, and were conducted in July and August, 2010. With the consent of participants, all interviews were audio-recorded.

Data Analysis

Each interview was fully transcribed and transcripts were made available to participants, who had the opportunity to provide corrections, additions, and omissions. Three participants utilised this opportunity to correct or clarify their record of interview.

In line with an inductive approach, thematic analysis was used to make sense of the data (Marlow, 2005). This involved the researchers examining the data to uncover recurring themes or what was collectively being said (Minichiello, Aroni, & Hays, 2008). Both authors were involved in this process and the findings reported reflect our shared understanding of the data.

Confidentiality is an important ethical consideration and confidentiality of participants in this study has been protected by ensuring they are not identifiable in any of the findings presented. Hence, names of participants have been changed, although information about their years of professional experience and the broad sector of their employment has remained as it was reported to the authors.

Findings

All participants had experienced social work to be stressful at times, and all reported periods of time when their desire to stay had been "shaken to the core". They also reported seeing "many good people drop away" from the profession, with Fiona expressing that she has seen many social workers "bash themselves up . . . and fall by the wayside". Nevertheless, they were all very passionate about their work and described feeling "lucky", "fortunate", and "proud" to be social workers.

Impact of Supervision

Supervision was mentioned by all participants as being important for their wellbeing and even "vital", either throughout their careers or at particular points. For example, Kate spoke of a growing appreciation of supervision from initially being an "adjunct or an addition" to her work, to the current time when it has become an integral, integrated, and more prioritised part of her practice. Several common themes centring on why supervision is useful emerged, with the most pertinent being its ability to act as a medium through which stresses and concerns can be externalised and explored. Supervision was thought to be useful in terms of facilitating critical reflection and as an important forum for learning. Other common characteristics of "good" supervision included regularity, discussion, and support. Kate also saw supervision as an important medium for generating constructive challenges and "working out where you need to improve your skills".

Early learning experiences or early mentors, or both, were still positively influencing and guiding the practice of participants. Both Alison and Fiona spoke of "still remembering" and utilising advice they had received from early supervisors. Dianne spoke of the benefits of having a "fabulous mentor" in the early phases of her career:

> Having a good mentor, supervisor, or role model there really helps . . . if you've got people you trust who are very honest with you. [My mentor] would say to me "Dianne, you need a challenge and I've set this up for you". And I'd go, "But, I don't want to do that", and she says "Bad luck, you're doing it". And I'd do it, because I'd been directed to do it, and it would actually be a really good thing. (Dianne)

Dianne also spoke of how a mentor can be useful in addressing one's weaknesses:

> You know, I often say to people, I'm very good at getting involved with a few different things and working and working and working and working. I actually need someone to say "pull back, you're getting tired and you've got to stop". (Dianne)

While appreciative of the potential positive impact of supervision, participants nevertheless acknowledged that supervision at times was far from ideal, especially the type of supervision that Thomas characterised as unsupportive, bureaucratic, and "tick and flick" in nature. A total lack of supervision at some stage in their career was also a common experience for the participants in this study. Fiona spoke of having experienced supervision as "often getting pushed aside in busy workplaces". She went on to describe how a lack of supervision early in her career had created a considerable amount of stress, and she gave the following advice:

> Having good supervision is really important, particularly when you are a new social worker. I think that is really important for that first 10 years-to set yourself up so you can be confident in what you are doing. If you are questioning all the time and you've got no-one to really bounce things off, how do you really know? And that is when burnout and stress comes in because you start questioning yourself and you think "Oh maybe I haven't done the right thing", "maybe I haven't done enough", "maybe I've done too much". (Fiona)

Line Management

For many social workers, professional supervision and line management are coexistent, with both roles being provided by the same individuals. Hence, in discussing their relationships with agency management, both Thomas and Kate specifically spoke of the importance of an "open door" policy; and said they have found that knowing they are able to have ad hoc and unscheduled discussions whenever they need to, is very important for their wellbeing. Thomas made the following comment:

> I know that I can go to anyone of my management colleagues and say, you know, "have you got a minute?", and just nut something out there and then. (Thomas)

In this vein, having "a good boss" with whom participants shared a mutual trust and respect and thus felt comfortable to speak to was considered very important. Fiona stated that she "couldn't work in a place where I had a boss whom I didn't trust or respect". Cathy mentioned that she found having a "flexible boss" who would let her "take off if I just need(ed) some space" to be very helpful in her management of daily stress. Nevertheless, an appreciation of the benefits of supervision did not necessarily translate into receiving formal supervision. This was particularly the case for the most senior social workers in their agencies, who were providing formal supervision to others but who were often not in receipt of any such support themselves.

Support and Informal Supervision from Colleagues

Whether or not participants had a formal relationship with someone who provided them with professional supervision, all participants spoke of the importance of the support and informal supervision they receive from colleagues. They experienced these collegial relationships as protective and as something that they can "fall back on". Common themes when talking about colleagues included support, teamwork, conversation, connection, constructive challenge, relationships, debriefing, and encouragement. "Bouncing off" another person and the support one receives from this type of interaction was a strong theme among the responses of participants, who all viewed this type of support as helpful in dealing with the stresses of the position. For example, Kate described collegial discussion as "quite critical" in "lessening stress":

> On days when you do feel really, "Oh, this has just been such a horrible day", those conversations are really important because they can say "well, you did this" and they can actually remind you of the stuff you have done. (Kate)

Others also spoke of the benefits they had experienced from having a strong social work department "behind them". A typical response included:

> For me, there is nothing like being in a social work department – where at times you can drive each other crazy but the support you get from your colleagues is terrific ... social workers are generally pretty nice people, so they are good colleagues, good people to be around. And I think being able to share with your colleagues is really important and being able to see that you are not the only one that might be feeling stressed or having challenges. (Fiona)

Dianne also specifically stated that she had derived benefit from having colleagues who are honest, who she can trust, and who can thus "keep an eye" on her, stating that "you can't always see [stress and burnout] yourself". Similarly, Cathy expressed having had colleagues "cover for her" and vice versa to be a useful strategy to "get time out" when she is stressed.

Professional Development

Professional development is a key aspect of professional supervision in social work and all participants commented on the important role of ongoing learning as contributing to their longevity in direct service work. All participants spoke of enjoying "updating themselves" and "expanding their horizons" by engaging with new literature and research, and stated that this has been particularly important for them in terms of their ability to remain engaged with their social work. For example, Thomas specifically expressed that ongoing learning was the main factor that has "kept his interest and enthusiasm very much alive". In addition to learning in the workplace, four participants had completed postqualifying courses at postgraduate level, with one holding a graduate certificate and three others holding their Masters degrees. However, it is unclear from these interviews whether there might be a link between further study and engaging in professional supervision; that is, whether further study is something that has been encouraged in professional supervision or whether in some instances it was embarked upon in the absence of an effective supervisor.

Discussion

This paper has explored the role of supervision in the professional lives of six experienced social workers, who considered themselves to be passionate about their work. In stark contrast to Saakvitne and Pearlman's (1996) suggestion that "caregivers are notoriously poor at self-care" (p. 61), participants in this study demonstrated a strong proficiency in terms of their own self-care, as well as an understanding of the importance of this aspect. Furthermore, the findings suggest that although they were experienced practitioners, they were not individuals who had "seen it all and could handle anything" without appropriate support, including professional supervision. Instead, a "seen it all and can handle anything" mentality can be an indication of the early stages of burnout (Brewer & Shapard, 2004; Guy et al., 2008; Halbesleben, 2008; Valent, 2002).

Just as there is no universal approach to preventing burnout among social workers (Dollard et al., 2001; Saakvitne & Pearlman, 1996), there is no one approach for promoting their longevity in the workforce. However, it has been suggested that social workers need to be supported in a number of ways, both individually and organisationally (Morrison, 2007) and that provision of professional supervision can contribute to the retention of social workers in the workforce, both at an agency level and also more generally to retain individual social workers within the profession. Whether or not retention of members in the profession was a rationale for the Australian Association of Social Workers (AASW) to include participation in supervision as a mandatory activity for accredited members is unknown (AASW, 2009), it could nevertheless have this benefit over time.

At an agency level, a lack of resources or the need to respond to ever-present crises can readily result in supervision not being prioritised by either social workers or agency management (Davys & Beddoe, 2010). While there will be times when rescheduling or deferring supervision is necessary and appropriate, such as in the midst of a crisis situation, agencies that value and prioritise regular professional supervision have a greater ability to retain social worker employees. Although it is often recognised that organisations need to pay particular attention to supporting new social workers (Vredenburgh, Carlozzi, & Stein, 1999), this study suggests that the guidance and support of an effective supervisor can contribute to staff retention, even for very experienced practitioners. In addition to providing support and guidance, especially in assisting individuals to recognise and respond to the emotional impact of the work (Figley, 2002; Guy et al., 2008), effective supervisors can also make a contribution to retention through encouraging their supervisees to undertake a variety of work (Morrison, 2007; Stalker et al., 2007), as well as have regular leave and holidays (Guy et al., 2008; Morrison, 2007), as well as develop other strategies for dealing with the stresses of the job (Saakvitne & Pearlman, 1996).

A strong sense of perspective was another key finding that participants emphasised as being closely related to their longevity in the profession and to which effective supervision could make a substantial contribution. In particular, a sense of perspective assisted participants in maintaining a mindset of autonomy, as well as a sense of accomplishment (Halbesleben, 2008; Russ et al., 2009; Stalker et al., 2007). More generally, it is recognised that a sense of perspective is essential in keeping one's role, responsibilities, and self-expectations both realistic and achievable (Guy et al., 2008; Kanter, 2007; Pines, 1993; Saakvitne & Pearlman, 1996).

All participants possessed a strong sense of curiosity and love of learning and they emphasised the importance of this in their longevity in the profession. Postgraduate education was common within the sample and opportunities for self-directed learning and critical thinking seemed important. Our findings suggest that to survive constant changes in both the profession and in the wider society, social workers need to be always learning (Kanter, 2004). However, the extent to which involvement in ongoing learning was fostered by supervisors needs further examination. While participants spoke of having had mentors early in their careers who had encouraged further learning, the role of supervisors in encouraging participants to enrol in postgraduate courses is unclear. Although there are many employing organisations that enable social workers to enrol in further courses of study, and facilitate this through the provision of paid study leave or flexible working arrangements that enable staff to attend university classes, individual supervisors or managers vary between actively encouraging supervisees to undertake further studies or passively supporting applications from staff.

One question that emerges from this study as warranting further exploration is the extent to which social workers embark on postqualifying courses of study as a consequence of either not having a professional supervisor in the workplace or not having a supervisor with sufficient expertise or experience in some aspects of the work. To this end, we note that for social workers who are members of the AASW, supervisory meetings that occur as part of academic study can be included in the requirements for supervision for accredited members of the association (AASW, 2009).

While the findings of this study support the proposition that professional supervision can result in the retention of social workers within the profession, the small scale and exploratory nature of the study, using a purposive sample of volunteers drawn from the researchers' professional networks, does limit the generalisations that can be made (Marlow, 2005; Rubin & Babbie, 2008). Culturally, the sample was also limited as by chance it included only individuals who identified themselves as Anglo-Australian and who spoke English as their first language.

It is also important to note that those interviewed were, in their own words, "survivors", and this study cannot answer questions as to whether or not personal characteristics such as curiosity or a desire for learning is more common in social workers who remain long-term in social work as compared to those who leave the profession. Nor do we know whether our participants' experiences of supervision, particularly early in their careers, were more favourable than those of their former colleagues who are no longer working in social work. Furthermore, participants in this study began their social work careers in a political climate very different from that of today (Dollard et al., 2001; Russ et al., 2009), and the extent to which the findings of this study might be generalised to new graduates entering the profession needs careful consideration.

Notwithstanding the limitations to the findings, if employers of social workers are looking to improve workforce retention and lower the costs associated with staff turnover, including replacement costs such as advertising for new workers and decreased morale for remaining workers, the provision of effective professional supervision is an effective strategy. Moreover, effective supervision should also improve the working environment and worker effectiveness for those social workers who are not currently seeking alternate employment (Mor Barak, Travis, Pyun, & Xie, 2009). While maintaining organisational commitment of social workers is not necessarily the same as maintaining a social worker's professional commitment (Coffey et al., 2009; Giffords, 2009), it nevertheless is an important first step in retaining individuals within the social work profession.

References

Anderson, D. G. (2000). Coping strategies and burnout amongst veteran child protection workers. *Child Abuse & Neglect, 24,* 839–848.

Australian Association of Social Workers [AASW]. (2009). *Continuing professional education policy 2009.* Canberra: AASW.

Brewer, E. W., & Shapard, L. (2004). Employee burnout: A meta-analysis of the relationship between age and years of experience. *Human Resource Development Review, 3,* 102–123.

Burns, K. (2011). "Career preference", "transients" and "converts": A study of social workers' retention in child protection and welfare. *British Journal of Social Work, 41,* 520–538.

Coffey, M., Dudgill, L., & Tattersall, A. (2009). Working in the public sector. *Journal of Social Work, 9,* 420–442.

Crisp, B. R., & Cooper, L. (1998). The content of supervision scale: An instrument to screen the suitability of prospective supervisors of social work student placements. *Journal of Teaching in Social Work, 17,* 201–211.

Curtis, L., Moriarty, J., & Netten, A. (2010). The expected working life of a social worker. *British Journal of Social Work, 40,* 1628–1643.

Davys, A., & Beddoe, L. (2010). *Best practice in professional supervision: A guide for the helping professions.* London: Jessica Kingsley.

Dollard, M. F., Winefield, H. R., & Winefield, A. H. (2001). *Occupational strain and efficacy in human service workers: When the rescuer becomes the victim.* Dordrecht, The Netherlands: Kluwer Academic.

Figley, C. R. (2002). Compassion fatigue: Psychotherapists' chronic lack of self care. *Journal of Clinical Psychology/In Session: Psychotherapy in Practice, 58,* 1433–1441.

Giffords, E. D. (2009). An examination of organizational commitment and professional commitment and the relationship to work environment, demographic and organizational factors. *Journal of Social Work, 9,* 386–404.

Green Lister, P., & Crisp, B. R. (2005). Clinical supervision of community nurses in child protection. *Child Abuse Review, 14,* 57–72.

Guy, M. E., Newman, M. A., & Mastracci, S. H. (2008). *Emotional labor: Putting the service in public service.* New York: ME Sharpe.

Halbesleben, J. R. B. (2008). *Handbook of stress and burnout in health care.* New York: Nova Science Publications.

Healy, K., Meagher, G., & Cullin, J. (2009). Retaining novices to become expert child protection practitioners: Creating career pathways in direct practice. *British Journal of Social Work, 39,* 299–317.

Kanter, J. (2004). *Face to face with children: The life and work of Clare Winnicott.* London: Karnac.

Kanter, J. (2007). Compassion fatigue and secondary traumatisation: A second look. *Clinical Social Work Journal, 35,* 289–293.

Kickul, J., & Posig, M. (2001). Supervisory emotional support and burnout: An explanation of reverse buffering effects. *Journal of Managerial Issues, 13,* 32–344.

Marlow, C. (2005). *Research methods for generalist social work* (4th ed.). Belmont, CA: Thomson Learning.

Minichiello, V., Aroni, R., & Hays, T. (2008). *In-depth interviewing: Principles, techniques, analysis* (3rd ed.). Sydney: Pearson Education Australia.

Mor Barak, M. E., Travis, D. J., Pyun, H., & Xie, B. (2009). The impact of supervision on worker outcomes: A meta-analysis. *Social Service Review, 83,* 3–32.

Morazes, J. L., Benton, A. D., Clark, S. J., & Jacquet, S. E. (2010). Views of specially-trained child welfare social workers: A qualitative study of their motivations, perceptions and retention. *Qualitative Social Work, 9,* 227–247.

Morrison, Z. (2007). Feeling heavy: Vicarious trauma and other issues facing those who work in the sexual assault field. *ACSSA Wrap, 4,* 1–12.

Pines, A. M. (1993). Burnout: An existential perspective. In W. B. Schaufeli, C. Maslach, & T. Marek (Eds.), *Professional burnout: Recent developments in theory and research.* Washington, DC: Taylor & Francis.

Pines, A. M., & Kafry, D. (1978). Occupational tedium in the social services. *Social Work, 23,* 499–507.

Rubin, A., & Babbie, E. R. (2008). *Research methods for social work* (6th ed.). Belmont, CA: Thomson.

Russ, E., Lonne, B., & Darlington, Y. (2009). Using resilience to reconceptualise child protection workforce capacity. *Australian Social Work, 62,* 324–338.

Saakvitne, K. W., & Pearlman, L. A. (1996). *Transforming the pain: A workbook on vicarious traumatization.* New York: W.W. Norton & Company.

Schaufeli, W. B., Maslach, C., & Marek, T. (1993). *Professional burnout: Recent developments in theory and research.* Washington, DC: Taylor & Francis.

Stalker, C. A., Mandell, D., Frensch, K. M., Harvey, C., & Wright, M. (2007). Child welfare workers who are exhausted yet satisfied with their jobs: How do they do it? *Child and Family Social Work, 12,* 182–191.

Valent, P. (2002). Diagnosis and treatment of helper stresses, traumas, and illnesses. In C. R. Figley (Ed.), *Treating compassion fatigue* (pp. 17–37). New York: Brunner-Routledge.

Vredenburgh, L. D., Carlozzi, A. F., & Stein, L. B. (1999). Burnout in counseling psychologists: Type of practice setting and pertinent demographics. *Counselling Psychology Quarterly, 12,* 293–302.

Australian Social Work Supervision Practice in 2007

Ronnie Egan

Social Work Unit, Victoria University, Victoria, Melbourne, Australia

Abstract

In 2007, a national online survey was conducted to investigate the practice of social work supervision in Australia. Six hundred and seventy-five social workers across Australia completed an online survey to produce the quantitative results reported in this article. The majority of respondents were female and were employed full time across a range of fields of practice, including statutory, non-statutory, and health and counselling settings. Nearly 84% reported having supervision. The largest number of respondents had received individual supervision in their place of work but some had also received more than one type of supervision. For more than two-thirds of the respondents, their principal supervisor was also their line manager, and most had had no choice in their supervisor. Despite the volume of supervision literature, there are limited empirical data about current supervision work practice in Australia. Findings from this study will lay a foundation for future research on social work supervision, a topic of significant importance to the social work profession.

Social work supervision is the process that socialises practitioners into the profession. Consequently, it is considered the cornerstone of professional practice. The dominant conceptualisation of supervision has been a professional one, where, within a supervisory relationship, three functions of supervision are undertaken: administration, education, and support (Fox, 1989; Kadushin, 1992a; Kadushin & Harkness, 2002). These three functions have been enshrined in the Australian Association of Social Workers (AASW) National Practice Standards for Supervision (AASW, 2000). The standards represent "a balance between agency resource constraints and ideal professional standards." The AASW, in line with other international professional social work associations, recognise the potential ethical implications of the organisational context on supervision practice. Scott and Farrow (1993) acknowledged in their research the "ambivalent place of social work supervision in the current context" (Scott & Farrow, 1993, p. 33). This "current context" refers to the managerial shift in the provision of human services driven by neo-liberal governments (Adams & Hess, 2000; Cockburn, 1994; Copeland, 1998; Daly, 2003;

Havassy, 1990; Hough, 2003; Laragy, 1999; McDonald, 1999; Morrison, 2007). Thus, the aim of this research was to investigate how social work supervision was practiced in Australia in 2007 within a managerial context.

The impact of managerialism has resulted in the states' resourcing of human service delivery becoming more dependent on measures of efficiency and performance measures, alongside an increased privatisation of human services globally (Jamrozik, 2009). The implications of the changes for social work supervision have been examined both in Australia and internationally. Australian studies by Wright (2000), Gibbs (2001), Clare (2001), and Lewis (1998) examined how the contemporary managerial framework of service delivery has negatively affected supervision, resulting in an increased focus on the administration function. Baglow (2009) and Clare (1991) suggested that there have been ambiguities regarding the norms and expectations of social work supervision, which has contributed to confusion about supervision practice directions both in Australia and elsewhere. Internationally, social work supervision practice has undergone radical shifts. In the UK, US, and New Zealand, supervisors have been licensed with accompanying mandatory training requirements (Cooper, 2006; Erera & Lazar, 1994; Froggett, 1998; Gibelman & Schervish, 1997; Kadushin & Harkness, 2002; Morrell, 2001; Munson, 2002). Other evidence suggested that managerialism has heightened the tensions between organisational requirements and professional responsibilities in the supervisory process (Beddoe, 2010; Hughes & Pengelly, 1997; Phillipson, 2002). However, despite this research some authors have argued that social work supervision remains uncontested and they have called for a closer examination of social work supervision practice in the current context (Hough, 2003; Ife, 1997; Jones, 2004; Noble & Irwin, 2009; Phillipson, 2002; Stanley, 2002). There is limited Australian research that has investigated how social work supervision was being practiced in the managerial context.

Research where empirical data about social work supervision practice have been collected has been largely international and has used surveys for large-scale data collection about supervision structure and content (Cooper & Anglem, 2003; Kadushin, 1974, 1992a; Munson, 2002; O'Donoghue, Munford, & Trlin, 2005; O'Donoghue, Munford, & Trlin, 2006). These studies have provided an indepth understanding about social work supervision practice. The only comparable Australian survey about social work supervision was undertaken in 1981, at the same time that managerialism was just beginning to impact on the Australian human service sector (Pilcher, 1984). At this time, Pilcher's results indicated that supervision was generally more available than it had previously been; considered necessary for effective professional practice; the quality was in need of an "upgrade," including more supervision training programs, and the professional association (AASW) needed to undertake a leadership role in this regard. Her findings were similar to those found in international surveys undertaken nearly 10 to 20 years later (Cooper & Anglem, 2003; Kadushin, 1992a, 1992b; Munson, 2002; O'Donoghue et al., 2005, 2006). The AASW has addressed one of her research recommendations in the development of the National Practice Standards of the AASW on Supervision (AASW,

2000) but it was unclear from the literature whether her other recommendations had been addressed. Research undertaken by Scott and Farrow (1993) investigated the extent to which supervisory practice conformed to the Standing Committee on Professional Supervision of the AASW's (Victorian Branch) Recommended Standards for Social work supervision in two fields of practice. Their results suggested that the standards were being implemented with limited differences across fields of practice. Such findings, alongside managerial changes to the human service sector, highlighted the need to increase current knowledge about social supervision practice and provided the impetus for the research reported in this article.

This was the first national survey about Australian social work supervision and, as such, provided an overview of practice. Data reported in this article were collected as part of a larger doctoral study. A mixed methods approach was used (Burke & Onwuegbuzie, 2004; Neufeldt, Beutler, & Banchero, 1997; Neuman, 2006). Both quantitative and qualitative data were collected and analysed to provide a picture of how social work supervision was practiced. It is beyond the scope of a journal article to present all results from this larger research project; therefore, this article focused on quantitative data about survey respondents and the structure of social work supervision as derived from the survey. The paper presents a picture of how social work supervision practice was structured in organisations in 2007.

Method

Design of the Study

Using an observational, prospective, cross-sectional study design, data about how supervision practice was structured within organisations in 2007 were collected. Structure refers to the types of supervision, a picture of who was supervising respondents, their location within organisations, and the nature of organisational arrangements supporting supervision. Resultant data were then used to build a picture about the delivery of supervision in the current context.

Participants

Three recruitment strategies were employed to access social workers from a diverse range of regions, sectors, and contexts across Australia. Advertisements about the survey and access to the survey weblink were placed on the front page of the AASW website, so that both members and nonmembers could access it, as well as being distributed via the internal email systems of Centrelink and the Victorian Department of Human Services (DHS) and in their professional newsletters. In addition, the survey was advertised via various professional meetings throughout Australia.

Measures

The Social Work Supervision Survey was developed, using previous Australian and international surveys about social work supervision (Cooper & Anglem, 2003;

O'Donoghue et al., 2005, 2006; Pilcher, 1984). There were two sections to the survey, the first for supervisees to complete and Section II for those supervisees who also identified as supervisors. Table 1 summarises the content of Section I of the survey. Items included open and closed questions with a range of response options.

Section II of the survey was for supervisees who were also supervisors. Items collected data about the length of time the respondent had been supervising; whether supervision was part of their job description; whether their organisation had a policy on supervision; numbers of supervisees supervised weekly; highest level of training in supervision undertaken and length of time since most recent training. In addition to the Social Work Supervision Survey, a data protocol was devised to collect information about the demographics of respondents. Information was gathered on gender, age, ethnicity, qualifications, work sector (Commonwealth, state, local, nongovernment organisations, and private organisations), length of time in current employment, employment arrangement (full or part time), and geographical location.

Once developed, the draft survey was piloted for face validity and user friendliness with 17 social workers (De Vaus, 2002). The 17 social workers included seven academic social workers and the remainder were Victorian human service managers and practitioners who had indicated interest in supervision and in the survey development. All social workers provided feedback during this piloting process. The feedback included suggestions about rewriting the introductory text; reducing

Table 1 Supervision Arrangements Survey Summary

Questions	Number of respondents
Part 1: Demographics of supervisor	
Gender	582
Age	582
Qualifications	542
Part 2: Organisational structures for supervision	
Type of supervision received (individual, group or both; Internal, external or both)	546
Most useful type of supervision received	173[a]
Supervision policies	584
Supervision contracts	576
Supervision as part of job description	584
Access to supervision	587
Frequency of supervision	574
Length of supervision sessions	574
Part 2: Location and feedback mechanisms of supervisors	
Internal and external location of supervisor	579
Supervisor as line manager	580
Choice of supervisor	581
Feedback from supervisor linked to performance appraisal	557

Note: The total number of respondents surveyed is 675, the reduced figures represent the missing data for each item

[a] The denominator here is 173 because it represents the subset of respondents receiving only one type of supervision.

demographic categories; reordering the initial sequencing of questions for respondents not currently being supervised; standardising language used in questions; clarifying ambiguous questions; changing the formatting; adding additional categories to some items; adding more items to the scaled questions; separating out questions which dealt with more than one idea; and changing the format for respondents skipping particular questions. These changes were incorporated in the survey design. A draft version of the survey was then trialled, reviewed, checked, and edited in response to the feedback from individuals participating in the pilot (De Vaus, 2002; Bryman, 2004; Cronbach & Shavelson, 2004) before being finalised.

Procedures

Ethics approvals for the survey were obtained from Victoria University, Centrelink, and DHS Victoria. Participation in the study was voluntary and information regarding this aspect was detailed on the first page of the survey. After this process, the survey was hosted online and went live in September 2007. When respondents completed the survey, their consent was confirmed online. An online format was chosen to collect descriptive data about supervision practice because it was cost effective, allowed for faster response rates, provided unrestricted geographical coverage, and left fewer unanswered questions (Bryman, 2004; De Vaus, 2002; McAuliffe, 2005; Rubin & Babbie, 2008).

Data were entered into SPSS (SPSS Ltd, Chicago IL) and descriptive statistics were generated to describe the group of respondents and the responses to the items on the Social Work Supervision Survey (Pallant, 2007). Levels of missing data on survey items ranged from 0.7% to 23.6% of respondents and Table 1 details this.

Results

Demographic Profile of Respondents

There were 675 respondents to the online social work supervision survey and 239 of these (29.5%) identified as both supervisor and supervisee. The majority of respondents (84.5%; 566/670) were women. Just over three-quarters (76.2%; 489/642) of survey respondents identified as Australian and 1.6% (10/642) Indigenous Australian respondents. The next largest ethnic group identified broadly as European comprising Irish, Scottish, Welsh, and European (13.1%). The remaining respondents (8.8%) were from culturally diverse backgrounds. Table 2 details the ages of respondents.

Undergraduate degrees were identified as the highest professional qualification (57.6%: 372/646) of survey respondents with a further (39.9%; 269/646) reporting postgraduate qualifications. To allow for anonymity, respondents were asked to name their employment sector and field of practice rather than their organisation. Table 3 details the employment sector of respondents as well as comparing it to demographic figures on employment sector available about membership (Northside, 2007). The

AASW membership figures use different categorisations of employment sector as noted which account for the specific differences across both data sets.

Most respondents (41.9%; 270/609) had been in their current place of employment for no more than 2 years. About another quarter (24.3%; 148/609) of respondents had been in their current position for between 2 and 5 years, followed by 17.1% (104/609) between 5 and 10 years and 14.4% for more than 10 years. The majority of survey respondents (78.1%; 479/613) identified as being employed full time, with 19.6% (120/613) employed part time, and the remainder were graduate students. Table 4 details the geographical location of respondents.

Section I, Part 1: Demographics of the Supervisors

Respondents were first asked about the demographic details of their supervisor, including gender, age and qualification. Over three-quarters (79.4%; 462/582) of supervisors were women and over the age of 40 (75.4%; 439/582). About 40% (39.1%; 212/542) of respondents reported that their supervisors had a minimum BSW qualification. Over a third (34.1%; 185/542) of respondents reported that their supervisor had a postgraduate qualification, and 18.8% (102/542) of respondents did not know the qualification of their supervisor.

Section I, Part 2: Organisational Structures for Supervision

Respondents were asked whether they were currently receiving supervision in the survey. If respondents answered "No" to this question, they were directed to continue the survey using their most recent supervision experience. The majority of respondents (83.7%; 507/606) reported having supervision. In terms of type of supervision, respondents were offered the following response options were provided: (a) internal individual supervision provided within their employing organisation; (b) internal peer group or facilitated group supervision provided within their employing organisation; (c) individual and/or facilitated group supervision provided externally and paid for by employing organisation; and (d) individual and /or facilitated group supervision provided externally and paid for by the respondent.

Table 2 Age of Respondents ($n = 675$)

	Frequency	Percent
Age		
20–29 years	157	23.7
30–39 years	175	26.4
40–49 years	157	23.7
50–59 years	149	22.5
60+ years	25	3.8
Total	663	100.0

Note: Missing data of 12.

Table 3 Comparison of Employment Sector between Current and AASW Data

	AASW AASW (2007)	Research Survey (2011)
State or local government	18.0	43.0[a]
Health, hospital, aged care	28.0	–
Commonwealth government	5.0	22.8[b]
Not-for-profit/NGO	23.0	23.6
Educational	8.0	5.8
Private (for profit)	14.0	4.8
Other – legal aid, overseas, justice, AASW	4.0	–
Total	100.0	100.0

Note: [a] includes health and hospitals; [b] includes aged care and disability
-Data not collected under these categories.

Almost two-thirds of respondents (62%; 310/546) had only one type of supervision, mainly provided individually in their place of work. The remaining one-third of respondents (30.9%; 154/546) reporting having two or more types of supervision, including a combination of either internal and external, group, or individual. When aggregating the figures about types of supervision, 71.6% had only individual supervision; 12.5% (68/546) respondents reported just having external supervision; and 15.9% (87/546) were having both types. Respondents were asked to identify the most useful type of supervision received. Almost half (46.2%;80/173) of the respondents receiving one type of supervision, identified individual supervision provided internally within their organisation as the most useful type received.

Respondents were asked about organisational policy on supervision, supervision contracts, supervision as part of the job description, access to supervision, and frequency and length of supervision sessions. Over two-thirds (66.4%; 448/584) of respondents had supervision policies in their organisation. Almost a half of the respondents (42.5%; 245/576) had verbal supervision contracts in place; almost a quarter (22.9%; 132/576) had written contracts; and over one-third (29.5%; 199/576) of respondents did not have supervision contracts in place. More than three-quarters (75.5%; 441/584) of respondents had an expectation of supervision in their job description. Respondents were asked if they had difficulty accessing supervision and one-third (38%; 223/587) reported having difficulty accessing supervision. Respondents were asked to indicate what were the contributing factors in accessing

Table 4 Geographic Location of Respondents ($n = 675$)

	Frequency	Percent
Capital city	349	57.4
Regional centre	190	31.2
Rural community	61	10.0
Remote/isolated	8	1.3
Total	608	100.0

Note: Missing data of 67.

supervision, including cost, time, inability to access appropriate expertise, no supervision provided in organisation, supervision not encouraged or valued in the organisation. Frequency of supervision was varied, as was the length of supervision sessions. Supervision sessions for 48.4% (278/574) of respondents were between 30 and 60 minutes. Table 5 details the data about supervision policy and supervision frequency.

Location and Feedback Mechanisms of Supervisors

Data were sought from survey participants regarding where, within the organisation, their supervisor was located; whether there was choice of supervisor; and feedback mechanisms in place for supervision. Respondents identified their supervisor's role in the employing organisation, internal or external to their team or organisation, or both. Nearly two-thirds of respondents (62.9%; 364/579) identified their supervisor as internal to their team; 22.3% (129/579) external to their team; and 14.9% (86/579) as external to their organisation. Further, respondents were asked a closed question about whether or not their supervisor was their line manager. For over two-thirds of respondents (67.4%; 391/580), their principal supervisor was also their line manager. Over four-fifths (81.6%; 107/581) of respondents did not have a choice of supervisor. Survey respondents identified whether feedback from their supervisor was linked to their work performance appraisal. About half, 50.4% (281/557) of respondents, had had feedback from their supervisor linked to their performance appraisal; almost one-fifth (21.5%; 156/557) had not; and less than one-fifth (17.8%; 120/557) indicated that they did not know if supervision was linked to their appraisal.

Section II: Supervisor Data

Section II of the survey collected data about those supervisees who also identified as a supervisor. There were 239 respondents who provided the subset of supervisees who were also supervisors. This section included questions about length of time they had

Table 5 Supervision Policy and Frequency

	Frequency	Percent
Supervision policy in organisation		
Yes	448	76.7
No	74	12.7
Don't know	62	10.6
Total	584	100
Supervision frequency		
Weekly	38	6.6
Fortnightly	162	28.2
Monthly	196	34.1
Quarterly	25	4.4
Sporadically	153	26.7
Total	574	100.0

been supervising and the supervision training were included. The data indicated an even spread across length of time they had been supervising, from between 6 months to more than 10 years. About one-third (32.3%; 75/239) of supervisors had undertaken "in house" supervision training, with almost one-quarter (24.1%; 55/239) undertaking training in the last 6 months.

Discussion

Results from this research present a picture of how social workers were being supervised across Australia in 2007. Over 80% of respondent social workers were supervised, with the majority receiving supervision in their place of work; and almost a third of these had two types of supervision, including internal and external supervision, or individually or in groups. So, despite other types of supervision being offered, the traditional individual supervision within organisations remained the dominant type of supervision provided, as well as being the most useful type of supervision. Almost 40% of respondents reported having difficulty accessing supervision. The difficulty in access related predominantly to time issues. On the one hand, the numbers of social workers having supervision was encouraging, while on the other, over a half of these are having difficulty accessing supervision. Further indepth analysis of the data are required to examine the nature of access difficulties and the rationale for more than one type of supervision.

An increase in the use of supervision policies within organisations was found in the current research when compared with data from almost three decades earlier, where "only two out of five respondents agencies had supervision policy" (Pilcher, 1984, p. 36). The value of supervision policies has been extensively documented (McMahon & Patton, 2002; Munson, 2002; Scott & Farrow, 1993). The literature suggests caution against assuming that organisations with formal supervision policies automatically translate into more effective or productive supervision experiences (Cousins, 2004; Scott & Farrow, 1993).

About two-thirds of respondents were supervised by their line manager and the majority of survey respondents had had no choice of supervisor. A review of the literature about line management and supervision in the managerial context demonstrated a greater focus on line management and organisational monitoring in supervision (administrative function), without necessarily valuing the other functions (Beddoe, 1997, 2010; Davys, 2007; Jones, 2004). Such reductionism towards managerial supervision risks breaking practice into small constituent parts and may not represent the nature of the day-to-day work or be influenced by supervisee's needs (Lewis, 1998). Line management has, in some cases, been substituted for supervision at the cost of other supervision functions, creating greater risk of blurred boundaries between managerial and professional aspects of supervision and an increased risk of authority being used coercively (Baglow, 2009; Beddoe, 1997; Beddoe & Davys, 1994; Cooper & Anglem, 2003; Gummer, 2001; Jones, 2000; Morrell, 2001; Stanley, 2002).

The AASW practice standards regard supervision in the social work profession as "going far beyond the concept of line management in administration and management" (AASW, 2000, p. 1). Most supervisees in this study were being supervised by their line manager. In a managerial context, these results have a range of practice, policy, and research implications. From a practice perspective, there is a need for transparency regarding the potential tension between the roles and responsibilities of line management and supervision. How this is translated into organisational policy requires an acknowledgement of these dual roles and the impact they have on accountability, conflicts of interest, confidentiality, contracts, performance appraisals, and finding the balance between the different functions of supervision. The way this is managed is a question for both the profession and for human service organisations. Research specifically examining the organisational conditions where the dual roles are compatible, and where they are not, would build on the current research.

A combination of both internal and external supervision was evident from the results. This finding was consistent within the literature, suggesting that there has been increased participation in external supervision (Bell & Thorpe, 2004; Cooper, 2000, 2006; Davys, 2007; Hirst, 2004; Itzhaky, 2001; Morrell, 2001; Ung, 2002). The reasons offered in the literature for an increase in external supervision were diverse and included the value of an outside perspective in supervision, introducing different perspectives, and separating the requirements of line management from the other functions of supervision. Given the increase in external supervision opportunities, how have practitioners embedded this into their practice? The implications of external supervision arrangements on social work practice and the value of using more experienced social workers in these roles requires more investigation.

Over a third of respondents indicated that their supervisors were over 50 years of age. The AASW has identified that the demographic of social workers aged 60+ years presents both membership and expertise challenges for Australian social work, due to the predicted numbers retiring from the profession (Northside, 2007). The available pool of supervision expertise will be affected by the imminent retirement age of the 60+ age group of social workers. Further inquiry into the numbers of supervisors in this age bracket may provide opportunities regarding the implications of the results for the provision of social work supervision in the future.

Limited supervision training options identified in this research were consistent with Pilcher's (1984) study. This probably reflected an enduring problem, given that access to supervision training for supervisors was identified as a concern in Australia in the early 1980s (Pilcher, 1984) and remained so in 2007. This stands in contrast to the training options evident in New Zealand, where supervision-specific training at both certificate and diploma level are offered (O'Donoghue et al., 2005). The AASW national practice standards for supervision identified minimum training requirements for supervisors (AASW, 2000). These include fieldwork supervision of social workers or the successful completion of an approved course in social work supervision or "post–basic training in a field of practice or method of intervention relevant to the supervisee's practice" (AASW, 2000, p. 4). Specific investigation regarding existing supervision training options and compliance with the AASW standards would provide insight about the barriers facing supervisors accessing specific training.

Limitations of the Study

Limitations of this research relate to representative sampling, online format of the survey, and the self-report nature of the survey. In the initial planning of the research, it was intended that a representative sample of social workers from the AASW database of 6222 members would be used (Northside, 2007), but AASW permission was not granted to do this. Therefore, the current research may not represent the Australian population of social work across different sectors, which impacts on the external validity of the results. The issue of representativeness of the sample is critical in relation to the capacity of these results to be generalised across different social work groups. The use of an online survey potentially created a bias towards respondents who were more frequent online users, often viewed as better educated, younger, and not representative of the general population (De Vaus, 2002; Bryman, 2004; Hewson, Yule, Laurent, and Vogel 2003). A further limitation is the current study is that data were based on self-report measures, and may have reflected respondents' perceptions rather than actual contexts or environment.

Conclusion

This article presented descriptive quantitative results from a national online survey on social work supervision in Australia. In a managerial environment, the empirical results from this research provided a picture of how social work supervision was structured in 2007, highlighting a range of variables that impacted on the structure of social work supervision practice. Some results relating to particular supervision training opportunities in 2007 remained the same as results from a Victorian survey on social work supervision undertaken almost three decades earlier. However, in 2007 differences were evident in relation to greater use of supervision, policies within organisations, and increased use of external supervision. Additional data sought in the current survey related to line management and its role in supervision and the implications of this in the current managerial context. Outcomes of this research have highlighted the need for further investigation into the structure of social work supervision.

Acknowledgements

The author acknowledges the social workers who responded so generously to the online survey in 2007. Without their participation this article would not have been possible.

References

Adams, D., & Hess, M. (2000). Alternatives to competitive tendering and privatisation: A case study from the Australian health industry. *Australian Journal of Public Administration, 59*(1), 49–59.

Australian Association of Social Workers (AASW). (2000). National practice standards of the Australian Association of Social Workers: Supervision, *Standing Committee on Professional Supervision.* Victoria.

Baglow, L. (2009). Social work supervision and its role in enabling a community visitor program that promotes and protects the rights of children. *Australian Social Work, 62*(3), 353–368.

Beddoe, L. (1997). A new era for supervision. *Social Work Now, 7,* 10–15.

Beddoe, L. (2010). Surveillance or reflection: Professional supervision in "the Risk Society". *British Journal of Social Work, 40*(4), 1279–1296.

Beddoe, L., & Davys, A. (1994). The status of supervision-reflections from a training perspective. *Social Work Review, 6*(5/6), 16–21.

Bell, H., & Thorpe, A. (2004). External supervision: What is it for a social worker in schools? *Social Work Review, 16*(2), 12–14.

Bryman, A. (2004). *Social research method.* Oxford: Oxford University Press.

Burke, J. R., & Onwuegbuzie, A. J. (2004). Mixed methods research: A research paradigm whose time has come. [Methodology]. *Educational Researcher, 33*(7), 14–26.

Clare, M. (1991). Supervision and consultation in social work: A manageable responsibility? *Australian Social Work, 44*(1), 3–10.

Clare, M. (2001). Operationalising professional supervision in this age of accountabilities. *Australian Social Work, 54*(2), 69–79.

Cockburn, G. (1994). Supervision in social work: A brief statement of the essentials. *Social Work Review, 6*(5&6), 37.

Cooper, L. (2000, July). *Organisational changes and social work supervision: Analysis and reconstruction.* Paper presented at the Supervision: From Rhetoric to Reality Conference, Auckland College of Education, New Zealand.

Cooper, L. (2006). Clinical supervsion: Private arrangement or managed process. *Social Work Review, 18*(3), 21–30.

Cooper, L., & Anglem, J. (2003). *Clinical supervision in mental health.* Adelaide: Australian Centre for Community Services Research, Flinders University.

Copeland, S. (1998). Counselling supervision in organisational contexts: New challenges and perspectives. *British Journal of Guidance and Counselling, 26*(3), 377–386.

Cousins, C. (2004). Becoming a social work supervisor: A significant role transition. *Australian Social Work, 57*(2), 175–185.

Cronbach, L., & Shavelson, R. (2004). My current thoughts on coefficient alpha and successor procedures. *Educational and Psychological Measurement, 64*(3), 391–418.

Daly, M. (2003). Governance and social policy. *Journal of Social Policy, 32*(1), 113–128.

Davys, A. (2007). Active participation in supervision: A supervisee's guide. In D. Wepa (Ed.), *Clinical supervision in Aotearoa/New Zealand: A health perspective* (pp. 26–42). Auckland: Pearson Eduction New Zealand.

De Vaus, D. A. (2002). *Surveys in social research* (5th ed.). Crows Nest, NSW: Allen and Unwin.

Erera, I. P., & Lazar, A. (1994). The administrative and educational functions in supervision: Indications of incompatibility. *Clinical Supervisor, 12*(2), 39–56.

Fox, R. (1989, March). Relationship: The cornerstone of clinical supervision. *Social Casework, The Journal of Contempory Social Work, 70*(3), 146–152.

Froggett, L. (1998). Sustaining tensions in practice supervision. *Social Services Research-Birmingham, 1,* 33–42.

Gibbs, J. A. (2001). Maintaining front-line workers in child protection: A case for refocusing supervision. *Child Abuse Review, 10*(5), 323–335.

Gibelman, M., & Schervish, P. (1997). Supervision in social work: Characteristics and trends in a changing environment. *Clinical Supervisor, 16*(2), 1–15.

Gummer, B. (2001). Abusive supervisors, competent workers, and (white) friends in high places: Current perspectives on the work environment. *Administration in Social Work, 25*(1), 87–106.

Havassy, H. M. (1990, March). Effective second-story bureaucrats: Mastering the paradox of diversity. *National Association of Social Workers, 35*, 103–109.

Hewson, C., Yule, P., Laurent, D., & Vogel, C. (2003). *Internet reserach methods.* London: Sage.

Hirst, V. (2004, October). *Growing social work managers through supervision.* Paper presented at the Global Social Work: Reclaiming Civil Society, Adelaide University.

Hough, G. (2003). Enacting critical practice in public welfare contexts. In J. Allan, B. Pease, & L. Briskman (Eds.), *Critical social work* (pp. 214–227). St. Leonards, NSW: Allen and Unwin.

Hughes, L., & Pengelly, P. (Eds.). (1997). Piggy in the middle: The place of supervision. In *Staff supervision in a turbulent environment: Managing process and task in front-line services* (pp. 23–39). London: Jessica Kingsley.

Ife, J. (1997). *Rethinking social work: Towards critical practice.* Melbourne: Longman.

Itzhaky, H. (2001). Factors relating to "interferences" in communication between supervisor and supervisee: Differences between the external and internal supervisor. *Clinical Supervisor, 20*(1), 73–85.

Jamrozik, A. (2009). *Social policy in the post-welfare state: Australian society in a changing world.* Frenchs Forest, NSW: Pearson Education Australia.

Jones, M. (2000). Hope and despair at the front line: Observations on integrity and change in the human services. *International Social Work, 43*(3), 365–380.

Jones, M. (2004). Supervision, learning and transformative practices. In N. Gould & M. Baldwin (Eds.), *Social work, critical reflection and the learning organisation* (pp. 11–22). Aldershot: Ashgate publishing.

Kadushin, A. (1974). Supervisor and supervisee: A survey. *Social Work, 19,* 288–298.

Kadushin, A. (1992a). What's wrong, what's right with social work supervision. *The Clinical Supervisor, 10*(1), 3–17.

Kadushin, A. (1992b). Supervisor and supervisee: An updated survey. *The Clinical Supervisor, 10*(2), 9–27.

Kadushin, A., & Harkness, D. (2002). *Supervision in social work* (4th ed). New York: Columbia University Press.

Laragy, C. (1999). Competition policies in human services: A review of employment services. *Australian Social Work, 52*(4), 39–44.

Lewis, S. (1998). Educational and organisational contexts of professional supervision in the 1990s. *Australian Social Work, 51*(3), 31–39.

McAuliffe, D. (2005). Putting ethics on the organisational agenda: The social work ethics audit on trial. *Australian Social Work, 58*(4), 357–369.

McDonald, C. (1999). Human service professionals in the community service industry. *Australian Social Work, 52*(1), 17–25.

McMahon, M., & Patton, W. (Eds.). (2002). *Supervision in the helping professions: A practical approach.* Frenchs Forest, NSW: Pearson Education.

Morrell, M. (2001). External supervision-confidential or accountable? *Social Work Review, 13*(1), 36–41.

Morrison, T. (2007). Emotional intelligence, emotion and social work: Context, characteristics, complications and contribution. *British Journal of Social Work, 37*(2), 245–263.

Munson, C. E. (2002). *Handbook of clinical social work supervision.* New York: Haworth Press.

Neufeldt, S. A., Beutler, L. E., & Banchero, R. (1997). Research on supervisor variables in psychotherapy supervision. In C. E. Watkins, Jr (Eds.), *Handbook of psychotherapy supervision* (pp. 508–520). Hoboken NJ, Canada: John Wiley.

Neuman, W. L. (2006). *Social research methods: Qualitative and quantitative approaches* (6 ed.). Boston: Pearson international.

Noble, C., & Irwin, J. (2009). Social work supervision: An exploration of the current challenges in a rapidly changing social, economic and political environment. *Journal of Social Work, 9*(3), 345–358.

Northside, P. S. (2007). *Australian Association of Social Workers (AASW): Membership trends and opportunities revisited*. Brisbane: Australian Association of Social Work.

O'Donoghue, K., Munford, R., & Trlin, A. D. (2005). Mapping the territory: Supervision within the association. *Social Work Review, 17*(4), 46–64.

O'Donoghue, K., Munford, R., & Trlin, A. D. (2006). What's best about social work supervision according to association members. *Social Work Review, 18*(3), 79–91.

Pallant, J. (2007). *SPSS Survival Manual* (3rd ed.). Crows Nest: Allen and Unwin.

Phillipson, J. (2002). Supervision and being supervised. In R. Adams, L. Dominelli, & M. Payne (Eds.), *Critical practice in social work* (pp. 244–250). Basingstoke: Hampshire Palgrave.

Pilcher, A. (1984). The state of social work supervision in Victoria according to the practitioners. *Australian Social Work, 37*(3), 33–43.

Rubin, A., & Babbie, E. R. (2008). *Research methods for social work* (6th ed). Belmont, CA: Thomson Higher Education.

Scott, D., & Farrow, J. (1993). Standards of social work supervision in child welfare and hospital social work. *Australian Social Work, 46*(2), 33–41.

Stanley, J. A. G., Chris. (2002). *In the firing line: Violence and power in child protection work.* Chichester, UK: Wiley.

Ung, K. (2002). The complex and diverse landscape of agency and external supervision. In M. McMahon & W. Patton (Eds.), *Supervision in the helping professions a practical approach* (pp. 91–104). Frenchs Forest, NSW: Pearson Education Australia.

Wright, F. (2000, July). *Supervision in the welfare marketplace.* Paper presented at the Supervision: From Rhetoric to Reality, Auckland College of Education, New Zealand.

Windows on the Supervisee Experience: An Exploration of Supervisees' Supervision Histories

Kieran O'Donoghue

School of Health and Social Services, Massey University, Palmerston North, New Zealand

Abstract

This article presents a qualitative study of New Zealand social work practitioners' experiences as supervisees. This study was part of a wider mixed-methods study of social work supervision. The aims of the paper were to explore how social work practitioners developed their understanding, participation, and use of supervision, and how their histories influenced their development and behaviour as supervisees. Sixteen participants were interviewed regarding their supervision histories. These histories were thematically analysed. Results showed that practitioners developed their understanding, participation in, and use of supervision over time. In addition, their supervision histories influenced their development and behaviour as supervisees both positively and negatively. These findings provide a starting point for further research into theorising about supervision from the supervisee's perspective and encouraging practitioners and supervisors to consider the influence that supervision histories have within their supervision.

The aims of this article are twofold: to explore how social work practitioners developed their understanding, participation, and use of supervision; and to consider how their histories influenced their development and behaviour as supervisees. This will be achieved through a literature review and a qualitative analysis of 16 social work practitioners' supervision histories. These histories were part of a more extensive mixed-methods study that explored the construction of social work supervision within New Zealand (O'Donoghue, 2010). The interviews referred to in this article followed a national survey of supervision practice (O'Donoghue, 2010; O'Donoghue, Munford, & Trlin, 2005). The research questions explored in this article are: What experiences influenced the participants' development, understanding, and participation within supervision as supervisees? And how did the participants' experiences influence their development and behaviour as supervisees?

Literature Review

The origins of the social work supervision literature date from the late nineteenth century (Burns, 1958; Kadushin & Harkness, 2002; Munson, 2002; Tsui, 1997a). Until the 1970s, this literature was concerned with supervisory practice, theory, and issues, and was composed of practice reflections, literature reviews, and theoretical ideas posited by experienced practitioners and academics (Munson, 1979; O'Donoghue, 2010; Tsui, 1997b). In the 1970s, efforts were made to develop the supervisory evidence base through basic descriptive studies of supervisory practice in specific situations (Chernis & Egnatios, 1978; Kadushin, 1974; Munson, 1975, 1979; Tsui, 1997b). Since the 1980s, research into social work supervision has been concerned with supervisory issues, namely role, relationship, responsibilities, interactional process, gender, and cultural differences, as well as the effect of supervision upon job satisfaction and client outcomes (Harkness & Poertner, 1989; Kadushin & Harkness, 2002; O'Donoghue, 2010; Tsui, 1997b). Critical reviews of this research undertaken by Tsui (1997b, 2004, 2005) noted that while several studies were concerned with supervisees' views and experiences, most examined their views about the availability, adequacy, and nature of the supervision provided, (e.g., Berger & Mizrahi, 2001; Gibbs, 2001; Pilcher, 1984; Scott & Farrow, 1993) rather than supervisees' understanding, participation, and behaviour. Barretta-Herman (2001) noted that limited attention had been given to the supervisee's role and contribution within supervision when she stated that there was very little written from the supervisee's perspective and said: "Little academic attention is given to the development of supervisees' skills and to full understanding of the purpose and process of the supervision relationship from the perspective of the supervisee" (p. 7).

A search of social work supervision texts published over the last decade (Austin & Hopkins, 2004; Davys & Beddoe, 2010; Kadushin & Harkness, 2002; Morrison, 2006; Munson, 2002, O'Donoghue, 2003; Shulman, 2010; Tsui, 2005) revealed that the literature specifically written for supervisees composed of instructional manuals, guidelines, and a report on a training course (e.g., Baxter & Mayor, 2008; Carroll & Gilbert, 2006; Davys, 2007; Inskipp & Proctor, 1988; Knapman & Morrison, 1998; Morrell, 2005). Generally, this literature attempted to address the lack of attention given to the supervisee's role, participation, and behaviour within supervision and provided practice wisdom designed to assist supervisees to construe and conceptualise supervision. From the literature searched, only Morrison (2006) noted the positive or negative influence that the practitioners' supervision histories have upon their level of engagement and participation. He also referred to the supervisee's contribution to their supervision history when he stated that, "the supervisee plays a part in the creation of his/her own supervision history" Morrison (2006), p. 88). It is this supervisee part that is the subject of this article.

Methodology

Participants and Sampling

Sixteen participants were purposefully selected from 52 respondents who expressed an interest in being interviewed as a supervisee, following the completion of a national postal survey questionnaire about social work supervision (O'Donoghue, 2010). Those selected were chosen from across New Zealand according to their location, field of practice, and type of supervision (all signalled by prospective participants in their expression of interest). The location criterion was employed to ensure that interviews were undertaken nationally. Likewise, selection on the basis of the field of practice was used to ensure that the interviewees reflected a range of the fields of social work practice. While the type of supervision criterion was intended to ensure that participants would reflect a cross-section of types.

The participants were predominately female (with only two male participants), aged between 40 and 69 years and mostly of Pakeha or New Zealand European ethnic identity (only 1 participant identified as Maori). The fields of practice that the participants worked in included health (6 participants), nongovernment organisations (NGOs) mainly child and family support services (5 participants), the statutory child welfare service (Child, Youth and Family) (4 participants), and a criminal justice service (1 participant). Their social work practice experience ranged from less than 5 years to more than 25 years, with the majority having 11 or more years of social work experience; 10 of the 16 held social work qualifications; and as a group they had had past experience of two or more of four different types of supervision (i.e., student placement, internal, external, and peer supervision).

Procedure

At the beginning of each interview the participants chose a pseudonym from a list provided and they were identified according to their pseudonym from that point on. They were asked to outline their supervision history from their very first experience through to their most recent experiences. In the process of reviewing their histories they were also prompted to consider how their experiences had contributed to their understanding of supervision and their participation in it as a supervisee. Towards the end of the discussion, each participant was invited to reflect on how they had developed as a supervisee over their career.

Data Analysis

Interviews were recorded and transcribed. Transcripts were reviewed and approved by participants prior to being analysed thematically, using NVivo, a qualitative research software program (see http://www.qsrinternational.com/). This analysis involved a close reading of each transcript and the identification of the themes and subthemes through coding at the respective nodes and subnodes. The data coded were checked by using the global search tool within NVivo. The interpretation involved moving beyond the NVivo analysis towards one in which the data were compared, contrasted, and explained in terms of their meaning. The study was approved by a University Ethics Committee.

Results

Supervisees' histories reflected each individual's experiences of supervision over time with different supervisors within various roles and organisational contexts. There was a notable difference between their initial experiences and those that occurred later when they had had more experience as supervisees. The results are reported in three sections; the first discusses the supervisees' foundational experiences, while the second explores themes present in their later experiences. The third section concludes with a brief discussion of the supervisees' reflections on their learning within the role.

Foundational Experiences

Participants' foundational supervision experiences were those they had had as students and in their first workplace.

Student Experiences

The supervisees' student supervision experiences revealed their initial understanding of supervision, their evaluation of the experience in terms of whether it was positive or not, and the influence this had had on their participation within it.

Among those for whom placement supervision was their first experience, a limited preparation and understanding of what supervision involved as well as an initial apprehension and anxiety about supervision were the main themes. For example, Belinda said she was "a little bit curious as to what it was..., but I wasn't really clear what supervision was all about." Whereas Joan, who was initially nervous, said: "[My supervisor] knew everything. And I was just a real dummy. So initially it was actually really scary. Even taking anything, I thought, well, this was stupid to take these nitty things to her because of her abilities..

Most referred to supervision positively due to the support they received from their supervisors and the learning they gained. For example, Barney described his supervisor as a role model who taught him particular skills that helped him develop reflective practice, professional safety, and to integrate theory with practice. Likewise, Hannah was also positive and said:

> The supervision was a lot of role plays, and it was brilliant. Absolutely brilliant! I learnt more in that because she would give me a case and we'd role play it. And she [the supervisor] was a very brilliant worker.

Felicity's experience differed from the others. She had felt unsupported and on trial and said:

I felt at odds with my supervisor ... and that was my first placement ... I'd felt so undermined by the whole process ... and I didn't really have the knowledge or skills at that time to actually understand what processes weren't supporting me ... It seemed ... there was something wrong with me, and I thought that I'm never going to make it in social work.

Not surprisingly, Felicity was nervous about supervision before her next placement. She indicated that this changed after a few weeks into her second placement, because she had felt supported and was able to discuss her experiences with two other students who were placed within the same agency. In other words, Felicity learnt that supervision could be different from her first experience through supportive experiences with another supervisor and the support of her peers. Felicity's experiences also illustrated how she had developed a mental map of the supervision relationship from her first experience and subsequently transferred this into her next supervision relationship. This mental map was then adjusted again as her perception changed as a consequence of the support she experienced in this second relationship. These experiences seem to agree with Hanna's (2007) assertion about the role that attachment theory and transference have in supervision and the need for supervisors to provide a secure base for supervisees, and aid their learning regarding how to act within this relationship.

Supervisees learning about supervision. As a group, participants learnt that the purpose and function of supervision was to support and assist their learning and to use the opportunity it provided. They construed it as the place where they reflected on practice, developed skills, knowledge, integrated theory and practice within an accountability and safety forum, in which they had permission to express, explore, gain understanding, and learn. Joan's illustrated this when she said placement supervision was:

About me as a person in my work practice... [and] was a very safe place to take issues ... a place where I could grow as a professional ... could be challenged on...some of my work practices. I could be challenged... and motivated enough to go out and bloody well put that [the practices] right.

Tamara typified the participants' learning about how to use supervision when she recalled that she had had to:

Bring what we were doing and discuss it in supervision with the person that would assist us in terms of developing our practice. A lot of journaling, videoing... We had to be prepared with the journal and ....sheets... that we had to do to bring to supervision.

Cara explained how she had developed her understanding of supervision and the supervisee role when she said:

I learnt what supervision was about...and I realised that I could bring myself into my work and use my own experiences to start informing what my practice was all about... But also learning that keeping that personal/professional boundary fairly clear ...understanding my own values system and what I was about and why I was a social worker and it made a huge difference.

The participants' experiences of placement supervision clearly inducted them into the practice of supervision to the extent that they understood its purpose and function, evaluated it in terms of whether it helped them or not, and were able to use it to assist their learning and development.

Workplace Experiences

All 16 supervisees spoke about their initial experiences within the workplace setting. For half, it was their first experience of supervision, whereas for the others it occurred after their experiences as students.

Those for whom it was their first experience were unqualified when they attained their first position and were employed prior to mid 1990s. The mid 1990s was when New Zealand social work began to professionalise, and the majority of employers required staff to hold social work qualifications (Beddoe & Randall, 1994; Nash, 2001). These participants' experiences varied from, not knowing what either supervision or social work involved and being very dependent on supervision, through to their experience being the ideal, which set the tone for their future supervision experiences. Keri exemplified those who had no idea what supervision involved. She said she was "chucked in at the deep end" with a supervisor who told her she would "either sink or swim." Her sessions were controlled by the supervisor who "would bring up whatever she thought was appropriate" and go "through caseloads... discussing what is happening in each case." There were no discussions about "supervision, contracts or what was expected from [Keri] as a supervisee."

Participants who came into social work from other professions recalled how they were dependent upon their supervision to provide them with the "knowhow" to work as social workers. For example, Odette, who came from a teaching, background said she was "totally dependent on supervision" to the extent that she was "going in all the time" to ask "what do I do now?" She described her supervision as "very directive and [it] needed to be." In contrast to the others, Carolyn described her first experiences as establishing the ideal for her of what supervision ought to be. She said it was "sacred for both of us, very developmentally focused [and] really very practical and pragmatic." It also gave her "good emergency support" as well as the sense "that you would always have that support." Carolyn summarised her experience as "really professional... humanitarian supervision... with room for challenge... lots of clarity and acknowledgement of what I was doing well and what I could do better." For these supervisees, their initial experiences provided them with instruction, support, learning, and guidance as they learned to become social workers and supervisees within their organisations. In addition, each indicated that their supervisors had played a key role in terms of leading, managing, and directing the supervision process. The success of the supervision process and the supervisees' learning clearly relied on their supervisors' leadership, facilitation, and support.

For participants whose workplace experiences followed their student experiences, supervision was focused upon learning to practice within their respective organisational settings. In some cases, it was concerned their client or casework practice, while in other cases it was about their roles and responsibilities within their organisations. For others, it had focused on their professional development. Abbey typified those for whom supervision was focused on casework. Abbey's supervision with her manager was "very much focused on how can I get through the next session with this client," with the supervisor's role being to "tell you what to do." Felicity provided an example of supervision that had focused on her role and responsibilities when she described it as concerned with "learning about the organisation" and being "clear about... the expectations ... and [her] job description." For Belinda and Joan, supervision had focused on their practice learning and development. In Belinda's case, she attributed this to her external supervisor, whereas for Joan this focus was due to the way her supervisor had challenged her personally and professionally and motivated her "to challenge myself a whole lot more, academically as well as professionally."

Taken as a whole, these supervisees' experiences mirrored that of the first experience (non social work qualified) group in terms of their supervision being work focused, instructional, and directive. They also experienced similar supervision types, with most having internal supervision and only one in each group experiencing external supervision. In addition, supervisors had a clear influence in shaping the process and focus of the supervision. Where social work qualified supervisees differed from the nonqualified group was that they had a deeper understanding of supervision and were more proactive in the supervisee role. They also did not express the same level of dependence upon their supervisors with their supervision being more focused on casework practice and their organisational role rather than their learning to practice as a social worker and learning to be a supervisee. Not surprisingly, the qualified social workers showed indications of a higher level of role development as both social workers and supervisees.

Overall the participants' learned from their foundational experiences to be supervisees and use supervision, with their supervisors socialising them into the supervisee role by instructing and directing them through the supervision process. Their experiences underline the role supervisors have in helping supervisees learn about supervision and how to use it, particularly when most participants reported not having a clear initial understanding of what supervision involved. Additionally, it also underscores the supervisor's role in helping the supervisee establish a secure base within supervision and a positive internal mental map of supervisory relationships (Hanna, 2007). It is with this in mind that one's attention turns to the supervisees' later experiences of supervision.

Experiences as Supervised Practitioners

Four themes emerged from participants' histories as supervised professionals. These were the influence of their development as practitioners, changes they experienced in their supervision, the influence of organisational policies and practices, and the effect of supervision training and becoming a supervisor.

Professional Development

Activities that were undertaken for participants' own professional development enhanced their understanding and use of supervision by increasing their knowledge, participation, and action in the supervisee role. Abbey illustrated this when she discussed how counselling and psychodrama training had influenced her as a supervisee by firstly considering herself and her reactions as part of the supervision process, and secondly through exposure to counselling models of supervision, particularly, Hawkins and Shohet's (2006) model, which she said informed:

> The areas I'm focussing on and so I might if I think I've missed something with a client... [or] I've been focussing on some area to the exclusion of others, I might try and deliberately take something else along to look at.

Abbey's professional development also contributed to her assertively seeking external supervision that would meet her needs. She describes this when she said:

> I have had to really fight to get this...supervisor. Because I wan-ted...supervision...that was more likely to be considering [the] thinking, feeling, action, aspects of a person's experience, of their social system, [and] of my own experience of working. And ...my self-development.

This link between professional development and an increased understanding, awareness, motivation, and participation in supervision was evident in all of the participants' histories. It was also apparent in a change in emphasis within their supervision whereby the supervisees' focus shifted from their clients to their professional practice processes. In short, the supervisees developed more awareness of the supervision process, a better understanding of their role as supervisees, and increased the level of responsibility they took for their supervision. This result is consistent with the argument made in the developmental supervision literature that there is a progression from a self-centred beginner, to client-centred novice, to process-centred professional, and then to process-in-context-focused advanced practitioner (Bernard & Goodyear, 2004; Hawkins & Shohet, 2006; Kadushin & Harkness, 2002; Stoltenberg, 2005). Moreover, it also indicates a need for further research into the relationship between practitioners' professional development and their knowledge, participation, and use of supervision as a supervisee. One possible implication of this in relation to supervisory practice concerns the degree to which supervisors take an active interest in encouraging their supervisees' professional development activities and aspirations, whereas another concerns how to facilitate improvements in supervisees' self-agency and ownership of their supervision through actively focusing on the supervisee's professional development.

Changes in Supervision

The second theme concerned how changes to the participants' supervision influenced their feelings, attitudes, participation, and use of supervision. All supervisees referred to how changes in their supervisor and type of supervision had affected them and their use of supervision. For some, these changes had had a positive progressive influence and led to them to personalising their supervision so that it would meet their needs. For others, the changes had had a negative effect on them as supervisees, resulting in their disengagement and deliberately reducing their level participation within supervision.

Changes with a positive influence. Changes that were viewed positively were those that involved: (a) securing supervision with a supervisor who was outside of their day-to-day work location; and (b) where they exercised a degree of choice or agency in relation to the supervision or supervisor. The consequences of these for the supervisees were that they used supervision more purposefully to meet their needs and they displayed a greater personal professional openness and trust in the process and relationship. For example, Abbey discussed how having an external supervisor after a number of internal field-specific supervisors, who were focused on cases, freed her "to explore relationship dynamics more, knowing that colleagues aren't seeing the same person or the problem isn't with the manager." She added that "[I could] look more at myself in terms of what I'm doing in my practice, what I'm doing in my relationships with other staff members" in a way that she could not in internal supervision. Likewise, for Joan changing from internal to external supervision resulted in her being clear about what she wanted from it. This resulted in her exercising greater self-agency and professional responsibility by advocating for her needs and ensuring her supervision contributed to her practice and practitioner development.

Changes that impacted negatively. These changes were those that resulted in inconsistent and substandard supervision. They also influenced the supervisees' level of engagement, participation, and motivation within supervision, because the supervisees perceived their supervision was not meeting their needs. Consequently, when faced with these situations and feeling insecure within supervision their behaviour became focused on self-protection in the face of what they perceived as a threat. Generally, it appeared that the supervisees' level of motivation, participation, and responsibility taken within supervision, mirrored the degree of acceptance of and satisfaction they expressed about their supervisor and the supervision. An example of this was Mandy, who became more discriminating and deliberate within supervision as a consequence of a tandem supervision relationship wherein she and another worker were supervised conjointly by the same supervisor. According to Mandy, she had had no say or choice about this arrangement, which did not work at all because she had had a "huge reaction to the supervisor and … fellow supervisee [and] … the quality of the guidance received around practical stuff … was not what I really wanted at the time." Consequently, Mandy spent "a significant period of time … being grumpy about those aspects rather than about the work."

Rima also had an unsatisfactory supervision experience. In her case, she had changed jobs and her supervision changed from external to internal with a team leader. Rima discovered early in this relationship that her supervisor was unable to deal with things that were emotionally challenging or of any substance when she experienced the following:

> [I] had to spend a lot of time on an incredibly distressed mother whose son was dying. They had just walked out and a man in front of them, committed suicide. That mother was so angry that anyone could take their life when she was fighting for her son's life, and I shared this with my supervisor. She changed the subject and I never ever shared another thing.

For Rima, this was "the most appalling supervision I ever had." She added that she had learned to "manage that hour so that I wasn't damaged" by working out "what not to say because I wouldn't get any response, or if I did it would only make matters worse." Rima only took superficial things to supervision sessions that:

> I probably know the answer to anyway and that would then lead on to ... to talk about how I was with the other services... So, in fact, I would initiate a conversation that I could sit and listen to for most of the time, which was really quite interesting, but really quite useless.

Hannah had also had a difficult experience, which occurred following a move from one office to another within the same organisation. Her change was from a positive experience of supervision in one office to another office where, "You had to watch your back." Hannah managed her supervision sessions by delaying her supervisor, by talking "about her children [for] the whole supervision ... then [would] come out and ... just do what I wanted." Explaining her behaviour, Hannah said: "I didn't have much respect for what she wanted done and so I did it my way, which sounds terrible!" In essence, the effect of this change of supervisor and supervision setting was such that Hannah had developed a defensive response to supervision, which meant that she avoided engaging in a supervision process.

Supervisees' responses to changes in their supervisors and supervision indicate that the interactional process with the new supervisors and context within which the changes occurred had had an influence upon whether the change was perceived and experienced positively or negatively. Notably, those changes perceived as positive and progressive were those that were agreeable and acceptable to the supervisees and those where the supervisee had a degree of say or influence upon. Whereas changes in the supervisor and supervision, where the supervisee seemed to have little influence and which did not meet their expectations regarding an appropriate interactional process and level of support, resulted in them choosing defensive strategies because they perceived supervision as unsafe and a threat. From the participants' comments, three areas of further enquiry arise. The first pertains to the supervisees' responsiveness to changes in their supervision, while the second concerns their emotional intelligence when faced with unsafe and threatening interactional processes. The third is about how might supervisees and supervisors work through such matters in an emotionally intelligent and professional manner (Howe, 2008; Morrison, 2007).

Organisational Policies and Practices

Organisational policies and practices affected the supervision of some participants through decisions made about the type of supervision, the availability, approval, and choice of supervisors. These decisions influenced the participants' motivation and behaviour within supervision in two ways. First, when organisational decisions enabled participants to take greater ownership of their supervision, be more proactive in their use of it, and participate fully in order to further their professional and practice development. In contrast, when these decisions increased the organisation's control of supervision, thereby reducing the supervisees' choices and options, participants were more reactive within supervision. Felicity, in particular, illustrated how a range of organisational decisions had affected her supervision. The first was when her supervision changed from being solely with a senior social work to a "two-tiered system" whereby she was accountable to a manager, while her clinical supervisor was another social worker. This arrangement, while adequate for reviewing casework, did not meet Felicity's professional development needs. Subsequently, she applied to have external supervision, which was not approved by the organisation. Therefore, she "ended up paying . . . for supervision" privately because she felt so strongly about it. Felicity said: "I saw supervision as . . . identifying my professional needs and I was going to go out and I was going to be proactive about meeting them. . . I knew I needed a different perspective." This external supervision soon replaced the internal social work supervision because her manager made a decision that her privately funded supervision met the organisation's requirements. The situation changed when Felicity was no longer able to fund the supervision and Felicity reported that "the organisation made it clear that it will not fund outside supervisors and they felt that there was enough skills and knowledge within the organisation to be able to do the supervision component for social workers."

Other organisational changes also occurred at this time. These included the establishment of multidisciplinary teams and the location of social workers within those teams, rather than as a team of social workers. According to Felicity, these affected supervision because the "access to other social workers to form those relationships [was] diminished," which limited the choices for a peer social work supervisor to someone that she would "meet on a regular basis." The peer supervision that resulted was described by Felicity as being problematic due to dual relationships resulting from "a limited pool of supervisors and being of that peer group and you're working with them and you're developing friendships." For Felicity, there was a gap between the organisation's policy that "we need to provide supervision for each other, [and the] practicalities of doing that," because, "the choices get cut down and your opportunity to have good quality supervision diminishes."

Supervision Training and Becoming a Supervisor

Supervision training was reported to be a factor that enhanced supervisees' understanding and participation in supervision, whereas the effect that becoming a supervisor had was mixed and appeared to depend upon the context in which it occurred.

Supervision Training

Abbey's comment that "my standard for what I wanted from supervision leapt up at that point. I want to be attended to very well, very closely. I want a supervisor who is up on that stuff" typified the views of the supervisees who had completed training in supervision. Like Abbey, other participants re-evaluated their supervision and became more motivated to act to meet their own needs and improve their supervision. Clearly, training in supervision aided both their understanding of the process and their motivation to have their needs met as supervisees. It also raised the question about whether there should be training provided for supervisees about supervision as part of continuing professional education.

Becoming a Supervisor

Almost half of the participants had previously been a supervisor. They all commented that becoming a supervisor affected their participation and use of supervision as a supervisee by changing their focus and how they participated and used supervision. However, there was a clear difference between those who had had line management supervisory experience and those who were peer clinical supervisors. Participants who were or had been line management supervisors noted that their supervision changed from being about practice to a focus on management tasks and staffing matters. In addition, their manager became their supervisor. Only a few believed this change was positive and identified improvements in their knowledge, understanding, participation, and proactivity within supervision. However, the majority reported a less positive outcome in which their supervision became a task and organisationally focused management meeting, with little or nothing specific to their development. For example, Cara received "very directional" supervision, with the consequence that she reverted "back to being directed ... and didn't challenge much" within supervision meetings. With the benefit of hindsight, Cara commented that her acceptance of this situation was one of the reasons why she had resigned from this position. The other participants' experiences, while not as extreme as Cara's example, also indicated that the supervision they had received upon becoming supervisors had inhibited their ability to take ownership of and be proactive within supervision and they reverted to receiving supervision rather than participating in it. The participants' experiences also raises questions about supervision by middle-managers and the extent to which the managerial line organisational culture shaped the supervision of these participants. Moreover, it indicates that the supervision of line management supervisors is an area in need of further research and evaluation, particularly given the majority of these participants indicated that their needs were not being met.

Those who were peer clinical supervisors had considerably different experiences from the line management supervisors. For instance, they did not change their job or supervisor as a consequence of undertaking the supervisory role. Instead, they continued in their current jobs as well as with their supervisors and added becoming a supervisor and providing supervision to their portfolio of social work practice. These participants commented that their supervisory role had helped them to become clearer about their own needs as a supervisee. This is illustrated by Rima's comment: "The more I made sure that their [her supervisees] needs were met, the more I realised how I would have to meet my own needs because they weren't being met here."

In summary, becoming a supervisor for the supervisees meant that their awareness was raised concerning their own needs within supervision and they gained an increased understanding of supervision. Whether or not this influenced their use and participation in supervision as supervisees depended on whether they became a peer clinical or line management supervisor and whether their supervision as supervisees was instrumental or developmental. Obviously, this suggests that the supervision of supervisors is an area for further research and evaluation, particularly in regard to the differences reported by the line management and peer clinical supervisors.

Reflections on Learning as a Supervisee

Most participants commented about their learning as supervisees. They generally noted that they had "grown" in the role and had given voice to the key things they had learned. For instance, Felicity, said that over time, "I have become a lot clearer about my expectations and of [them] being met." She added that "I am not as accepting if it's not working." Noting that she had learnt "how supervision works, what it's about, how to get the best out of supervision ... the opportunities that it provides, the barriers to good supervision ... to be proactive in getting a model of supervision that works best." Tamara also commented that through her past supervision experiences she had become "very clear what my needs are and [was] not afraid to ask for them... [as well as] make sure they get met." Therefore, participants' understandings and practices within the supervisee role had evolved over time to the point where it involved an increased awareness of the supervision process, the supervisee role, and their own needs, together with the motivation to pursue proactively those needs with confidence within the supervision forum.

Discussion

A constant theme across most of the supervisees' histories was that over time there was a progressive journey from being supervised, to the supervision of client practice, through to supervision as a professional practitioner (Bernard & Goodyear, 2004; Hawkins & Shohet, 2006; Kadushin & Harkness, 2002; Stoltenberg, 2005). Changes that occurred in their behaviour and use of supervision during this process progressed from receiving instruction and responding to questions and direction; bringing and discussing clients and client-related issues; through to actively utilising supervision to develop their professional practice and meet their needs as practitioners. Contributing factors in the supervisees' progress were safe and secure foundational experiences with a supervisor, who was a secure base and who inducted them into their roles and into the process. Following this foundational experience, the journey continued through supervisees' professional development experiences, positively viewed changes in their supervision and supervisor, supervision training, and in becoming a peer clinical supervisor. In a number of cases, supervisees' growth within supervision involved securing external supervision or a supervisor that the supervisee had chosen. Supervisees' growth and development within supervision was signposted by increases in their participation, motivation, ownership, and proactivity (Bernard & Goodyear, 2004; Hawkins & Shohet, 2006; Kadushin & Harkness, 2002; Stoltenberg, 2005). This journey from "being supervised" to "my supervision" was not a linear progression; rather, it involved a number of turns, sharp corners, and occasional dead ends. This was particularly evidenced among supervisees whose use and participation in supervision regressed, where they had actively disengaged and subverted the process to protect themselves from perceived threat. Generally, this occurred when their expectations of the interactional process were not met and they had little choice regarding supervision or supervisor. It was notable that this primarily occurred within internal line management supervision relationships. A related finding was that supervisees who were or had been line management supervisors were also inhibited; however, in their case, instead of disengaging and subverting the process they reverted to the stage of being instructed and directed within supervision.

Implications of this Research

A number of implications arise from the participants' supervision histories. The first and most obvious implication concerns the transferability of the supervision experiences of participants in this study to other supervisees and practitioners, and the extent to which these experiences resonate with them or raise questions about: (a) whether their own needs are being met within supervision; (b) their degree of use and participation in supervision; and (c) their own growth and developmental journeys within the supervisee role. In addition, participants' histories also showed the importance for supervisees of being informed about supervision and how to use it, as well as assertively voicing their needs and expectations (Barretta-Herman, 2001; Carroll & Gilbert, 2006; Davys, 2007, Inskipp & Proctor, 1988; Knapman & Morrison, 1998; Morrell, 2005). This is particularly significant, as O'Donoghue (2010) pointed out, because notions of responsibility within supervision are shifting from organisations and supervisors to practitioners, who are now seen to have an ethical responsibility and statutory direction to participate in supervision (e.g., Aotearoa New Zealand Association of Social Workers, 2008; Social Workers Registration Board, 2006). In other words, when faced with inadequate and unsafe supervision, supervisees may find themselves in difficult circumstances if they actively disengage and subvert their supervision process. There is an obvious need to develop supervisees' emotionally intelligent and problem-solving strategies so that when they are faced with unsafe and threatening interactions they know how to work these through professionally (Morrison, 2007).

Implications for supervisory practice focus attention on how supervisors can assist their supervisees, and understand, use, and make the most of supervision (Brown & Bourne, 1996; Morrison, 2006). When working with beginning supervisees, the message clearly concerns inducting and teaching them how to use supervision, while at the same time providing the safe secure base for supervisees to construct a positive mental map of supervision and supervisory relationships (Hanna, 2007). For experienced and established practitioners, the challenge seems to be to connect their professional development interests with their supervision and to encourage them to view everything that they bring to supervision within this context (Davys & Beddoe, 2010). There are also implications for starting new relationships, where the supervisee has had to change supervisor and has had limited options or voice in this process. In such cases, it is important for the supervisor to explore the supervisees' history and feelings about the change in supervision arrangements and to attend assiduously to the supervisee during the interactional process (Shulman, 2010).

Implications for managers arising from the supervisees' histories relate to the supervision provided to line management supervisors and how to enhance the professional development aspects as well as the interactional processes, and to consider the need for external supervision for supervisors where this cannot be provided within the managerial line (Hirst, 2001). With regard to organisational policies and practices related to supervision, the message from participants concerned opportunities and options available to them and the overall importance of supervision for their ongoing professional development (Jones, 2004). Another message from the findings of this study is that when the level of surveillance, control, and risk management within supervision was increased it was arguably counter-productive because of the effect it had in reducing supervisees' participation and ownership of their supervision (Beddoe, 2010).

Limitations of the Study

A limitation of this exploratory study was that data were derived from 16 supervisees recalled accounts of their supervision history, thereby relying on the credibility of the participants, their recollections, and the interpretation of participants' responses by the researcher (Patton, 2002). This means that the transferability of findings and claims made are limited to the extent to which these resonate with or raise questions for readers in terms of their own supervision experiences and contexts (Fook, 2002).

Clearly, there is a need for further research regarding supervisees' perspectives, experiences, roles, participation in, and behaviour within supervision. Throughout this article, areas for further research have been identified in regard to: (a) factors that contribute to the development of a secure base within supervision; (b) the link between professional development and supervisee participation, ownership, motiva-tion, and proactivity; (c) the extent to which choice and the availability of supervision outside of one's workplace impact upon the capacity of supervisees to make the most of their supervision; (d) how changes in supervision affect supervisees; (e) how supervisees can respond in an emotionally intelligent and professional way to supervision they perceive as inadequate and unsafe; and (f) line managers experiences of supervision as supervisees. In summary, there is a significant research agenda with regard to supervisees' experiences within supervision and their management of these experiences within the professional role-set and expectations of being a social work supervisee.

Conclusion

The aims of this article were to explore how social work practitioners developed their understanding, participation in, and use of supervision as supervisees; and to examine how their histories influenced their development and behaviour as supervisees. With regard to the first aim, results have shown that participants developed their understanding, participation, and use of supervision through their foundational experiences and through their ongoing professional development, as well as through the changes they experienced in their supervision over time. In relation to the second aim, participants' histories did influence their development and behaviour as supervisees, with the experiences they perceived as positive leading to increased participation, motivation, ownership, and proactivity; whereas experiences that they perceived negatively resulted in them adopting behaviours that enabled them to disengage, subvert or manage the perceived threat that supervision posed, or revert to receiving supervision and being instructed by their supervisor. In conclusion, the results and discussion in this paper provide a starting point for further research into the conceptualisation of and theorising about supervision from the perspective of supervisees. These results also encourage practitioners and supervisors to consider the influence that supervision histories, interactional processes, and supervision context have on supervisees' participation and behaviour within supervision.

References

Aotearoa New Zealand Association of Social Workers. (2008). *Code of ethics*. Christchurch, New Zealand: ANZASW.

Austin, M., & Hopkins, K. (Eds.). (2004). *Supervision as collaboration in the human services: Building a learning culture*. Thousand Oaks, CA: Sage.

Barretta-Herman, A. (2001). Fulfilling the commitment to competent social work practice through supervision. In L. Beddoe & J. Worrall (Eds.), *Supervision conference from rhetoric to reality: Keynote address and selected papers* (pp. 1–10). Auckland, New Zealand: Auckland College of Education.

Baxter, R., & Mayor, T. (2008). *Supervision scrapbook*. Wellington: Authors.

Beddoe, L. (2010). Surveillance or reflection: Professional supervision in 'the risk society'. *British Journal of Social Work*, 40(4), 1279–1296.

Beddoe, L., & Randal, H. (1994). The New Zealand Association of Social Workers: The professional response to a decade of change. In R. Munford & M. Nash (Eds.), *Social work in action* (pp. 21–36). Palmerston North, New Zealand: Dunmore Press.

Berger, C., & Mizrahi, T. (2001). An evolving paradigm of supervision within health care environments. *Social Work in Health Care, 32*(4), 1–18.

Bernard, J., & Goodyear, R. (2004). *Fundamentals of clinical supervision* (3rd ed.). Boston: Allyn &Bacon.

Brown, A., & Bourne, I. (1996). *The social work supervisor: Supervision in community, day care, and residential settings.* Buckingham, UK: Open University Press.

Burns, M. (1958). *The historical development of the process of casework supervision as seen in the professional literature of social work.* Unpublished PhD dissertation, The University of Chicago, Ann Arbor, MI, University Microfilms International.

Carroll, M., & Gilbert, M. (2006). *On being a supervisee: Creating learning partnerships.* Kew, Victoria: PsychOz.

Chernis, C., & Egnatios, E. (1978). Clinical supervision in community mental health. *Social Work, 23*(3), 219–223.

Davys, A. (2007). Active participation in supervision: A supervisee's guide. In D. Wepa (Ed.), *Clinical supervision in Aotearoa New Zealand: A health perspective* (pp. 26–42). Auckland: Pearson Education.

Davys, A., & Beddoe, L. (2010). *Best practice in professional supervision: A guide for the helping professions.* London: Jessica Kingsley.

Fook, J. (2002). Theorizing from practice: Towards an inclusive approach for social work research. *Qualitative Social Work, 1*(1), 79–95.

Gibbs, J. (2001). Maintaining front-line workers in child protection: A case for refocusing supervision. *Child Abuse Review, 10*, 323–335.

Hanna, S. (2007). Not so strange! An application of attachment theory and feminist psychology to social work supervision. *Aotearoa New Zealand Social Work Review, 19*(3), 12–22.

Harkness, D., & Poertner, J. (1989). Research and social work supervision: A conceptual review. *Social Work, 34*(2), 115–119.

Hawkins, P., & Shohet, R. (2006). *Supervision in the helping professions* (3rd ed.). Maidenhead, Berkshire, UK: Open University Press.

Hirst, V. (2001). *Professional supervision for managers: An effective organisational development intervention: an inquiry based on the perceptions and experiences of managers of social work.* Unpublished Masters thesis, University of Auckland, Auckland, New Zealand.

Howe, D. (2008). *The emotionally intelligent social worker.* Basingstoke, Hampshire: Palgrave.

Inskipp, F., & Proctor, B. (1988). *Skills for supervising and being supervised.* St. Leonards on Sea, East Sussex: Alexia Publications.

Jones, M. (2004). Supervision, learning and transformative practices. In N. Gould & M. Baldwin (Eds.), *Social work, critical reflection and the learning organization* (pp. 11–22). Burlington, VT: Ashgate.

Kadushin, A. (1974). Supervisor-supervisee: A survey. *Social Work, 19*(3), 288–298.

Kadushin, A., & Harkness, D. (2002). *Supervision in social work* (4th ed.). New York: Columbia University Press.

Knapman, J., & Morrison, T. (1998). *Making the most of supervision in health and social care: A self-development manual for supervisees.* Brighton, UK: Pavilion.

Morrell, M. (2005). Supervision an effective partnership: The experience of running workshops for supervisees in 2004–5. *Social Work Review, 17*(4), 39–45.

Morrison, T. (2006). *Staff supervision in social care: Making a real difference for staff and service users* (3rd ed.). Brighton, UK: Pavilion.

Morrison, T. (2007). Emotional intelligence, emotion and social work: Context, characteristics, complications and contribution. *British Journal of Social Work, 37*(2), 245–263.

Munson, C. (1975). *The uses of structural, authority and teaching models in social work supervision.* Unpublished DSW dissertation, University of Maryland, Ann Arbor, MI, University Microfilms International.

Munson, C. (1979). Authority and social work supervision: An emerging model. In C. Munson (Ed.), *Social work supervision: Classic statements and critical issues* (pp. 336–346). New York: Free Press.

Munson, C. (2002). *Handbook of clinical social work supervision* (3rd ed.). Binghamton, NY: Haworth Social Work Practice.

Nash, M. (2001). Social work in Aotearoa New Zealand: Its origins and traditions. In M. Connolly (Ed.), *New Zealand social work: Context and practice* (pp. 32–43). Auckland, New Zealand: Oxford University Press.

O'Donoghue, K. (2003). *Restorying social work supervision.* Palmerston North, New Zealand: Dunmore.

O'Donoghue, K. (2010). *Towards the construction of social work supervision in Aotearoa New Zealand: A study of the perspectives of social work practitioners and supervisors.* PhD thesis, Massey University, Palmerston North.

O'Donoghue, K., Munford, R., & Trlin, A. (2005). Mapping the territory: Supervision within the Association. *Social Work Review, 17*(4), 46–64.

Patton, M. (2002). *Qualitative research and evaluation methods* (3rd ed). Thousand Oaks, CA: Sage.

Pilcher, A. J. (1984). The state of social work supervision in Victoria according to the practitioners. *Australian Social Work, 37*(3/4), 33–43.

Scott, D., & Farrow, J. (1993). Evaluating standards of social work supervision in child welfare and hospital social work. *Australian Social Work, 46*(2), 33–41.

Shulman, L. (2010). *Interactional supervision* (3rd ed). Washington, DC: NASW Press.

Social Workers Registration Board. (2006). *Code of conduct guidelines.* Retrieved September 10, 2011 from http://www.swrb.govt.nz/files/CodeofConduct/CodeOfConductGuidelines_Aug08.pdf.

Stoltenberg, C. (2005). Enhancing professional competence through developmental approaches to supervision. *American Psychologist, 60*(8), 857–864.

Tsui, M. (1997a). The roots of social work supervision: An historical review. *The Clinical Supervisor, 15*(2), 191–198.

Tsui, M. (1997b). Empirical research on social work supervision: The state of the art (1970–1995). *Journal of Social Service Research, 23*(2), 39–54.

Tsui, M. (2004). Charting the course of future research on supervision. In M. Austin & K. Hopkins (Eds.), *Supervision as collaboration in the human services: Building a learning culture* (pp. 272–280). Thousand Oaks, CA: Sage.

Tsui, M. (2005). *Social work supervision: Contexts and concepts.* Thousand Oaks, CA: Sage.

Social Work Supervision for Changing Contexts

Liz Beddoe

School of Counselling, Human Services and Social Work, University of Auckland, Auckland, New Zealand

Abstract

Internationally many social work professional bodies require practitioners to participate in regular clinical supervision. Supervision is believed to support continuing development of professional skills, the safeguarding of competent and ethical practice and oversight of the wellbeing of the practitioner. This chapter considers what might be needed over the stages of social workers' careers and explores some aspects of diversity in the modes of delivery of supervision, including supervision between members of different professions.

Supervision in the Age of Austerity

In 2013 Jane Wonnacott presented a conference paper entitled "*Supervision: A luxury or critical to good practice in times of austerity*" and noted:

> As cuts bite, we could be heading for a perfect storm – as families face increased hardship, child protection workers are likely to be dealing with ever more complex problems with a reduction in external resources at the same time as they are being asked to move beyond a compliance based model of practice. (2013, p.13)

In spite of funding cuts, supervision has been retained as a core practice in social work. Baines, Charlesworth, Turner and O'Neill (2014) recently researched the changing workplace relations and the experiences of social workers in the non-profit sector in Canada, Australia, Scotland and New Zealand. Among their findings was the evidence that within the managerialist environment and challenging economic conditions the "agency's mission, supportive supervision" and the workers' commitment to the communities they served were highly significant. Such features operated to buffer "the negative impacts of NPM and other forms of managerialism, providing spaces in which workers can express their values on the job and reinforce their sense of themselves as linked to larger moral or social justice projects" (Baines et al., 2014, p. 3). Supervision thus offers an important mediating role in supporting practitioners to remain "on mission" during stressful times of constraint and intense scrutiny. Drawing together themes from the reporting of many reviews of practice, Wonnacott emphasises the enduring importance of supervision:

> In this age of austerity we cannot afford *not* to supervise effectively. When we are struggling with scarce resources and dealing with ever more complex problems we need to foster resilience by providing front line staff with the scaffolding they need to get out there, work with the most vulnerable members of our society with the

emotional intelligence and compassion that will make a difference. (Wonnacott, 2013, p. 15)(Emphasis added)

While such a case is often made that supervision is essential for safe, accountable social work practice it is not entirely accepted without contest that supervision is effective, nor is it a universal activity. While reflective clinical supervision is strongly promoted over managerial supervision (Noble & Irwin, 2009), concern is also expressed that we need reliable evidence that supervision does what it is supposed to. This is neatly summed up in the following passage: "Needless to say, supporters and critics of supervision all argue for the revitalization of supervision. But, is the faith in supervision justified? What are the outcomes it can be expected to achieve?" (Carpenter, Webb & Bostock, 2013, p. 1843). While acknowledging that the case for supervision is empirically weak, reflecting on the findings of their review of the supervision research literature Webb et al. (2013, p. 1851) suggest that there is some empirical support for the following claims:

- "Supervision works best when it pays attention to task assistance, social and emotional support and a positive interpersonal relationship between supervisors and supervisees";
- "Given the evidence that supervision is associated with job satisfaction and protects against stress, practitioners should insist that good supervision be provided by their employers";
- Supervision should move beyond a task focus to "providing opportunities for reflective supervision";
- "Effective supervision is an important element of an organization's duty of care to its employees, and to the consumers it serves";
- "Effective supervision is associated with more positive perceptions of job performance and a greater ability to manage workloads, while employees' case analysis and planning skills are honed".

These findings are important as supervision is an expensive activity, taking workers away from direct work with service users, and inevitably questions will be asked about whether supervision should be directed to those most in need. Bearing such a challenge in mind two linked themes can be usefully explored in this chapter: firstly, are there different supervision requirements throughout the career of the social worker? The second theme considers the potential gains and challenges offered by the growing practice of interprofessional supervision.

Supervision as a Feature of Social Work Careers

It seems well established in social work that supervision is a long term practice within social work careers. Hair (2013, p. 1565) notes an "enduring belief that practice-focused supervision is needed throughout the career of the social worker". Many professional associations and/or regulatory bodies provide policy and guidance to outline what are the minimum supervision requirements as noted in Table 1 below. However, as Hair points out these bodies "are silent about an end point for supervision" (2013, p. 1565). Table 1 lists the requirements for supervision and related information gathered from selected jurisdictions. While most set some guidelines regarding frequency for new graduates and this is often linked to requirements for continuing development, registration or licensing, the policies do not suggest an end-point. It is almost always mandatory that supervision will be provided by a qualified social worker.

Despite an assumption that supervision should be eternal, the literature does provide some contrary opinions on the importance of lifelong supervision for practitioners in social work. Laufer (2004, p. 154) reviewed the literature and found several earlier arguments challenging lifelong supervision including some opinion that continuing supervision might "damage the profession and its prestige" (Mandell, 1979; Veeder, 1991). Supervision in social work has been criticized for fostering dependency with consequences for the status of the profession (Veeder, 1991). From this perspective it is felt that "autonomy and professionalism mean the ability to work and make decisions without dependency on factors such as intensive supervision" (Laufer, p. 154). The advantages of supervision are thus believed to be time-limited, contributing less as the practitioner matures. Laufer notes that supervision in its current form was developed before formal social work education was well-established and supervision was the way of learning and training new workers in an apprenticeship model.

Table 1 Supervision Requirements in Selected Countries

Professional body/regulator	Supervision requirements	Links to licensing and ongoing professional development
AASW	Supervision required and liked to CPD.	The AASW recommends that social workers access supervision from experienced social work practitioners however acknowledges that some social workers choose to access external supervision from professionals other than social workers. Also acknowledges that some social workers are often supervised by other allied professionals in agency contexts.
ANZASW/ SWRB	To meet the supervision standards of competency, all ANZASW members in practise are required to be engaged in core social work supervision for at least one hour per month. It is anticipated that most members will have additional requirements for supervision. In the first year of practice ANZASW members are required to have a minimum of one-hour core social work supervision per week.	The Social Workers Registration Act does not specify an expectation for supervision although Section 29 (1) & (2) outlines that the Board may adopt conditions for practising certificates that may include supervision. Supervision is . . . considered by the Board to be an essential element ensuring competent social work practice. Attestation needed for Annual Practising Certificate (SWRB, 2013)

ASWB/ NASW	There is countrywide agreement that time-limited, post-degree, practice focused supervision is needed, the duration of expected supervision is variable by state and can range from 75–200 hours completed over 2–3 years. (Association of Social Work Boards ASWB), 2006–12). (ASWB 2009)	The NASW (2005,p.16) delineates the amount of clinical supervision required for clinical social workers, from regular 'professional social work supervision' for practitioners with less than five years of practice experience to 'consultation on an as-needed, self-determined basis' for clinicians with five years or more of experience'.
BASW	Receive regular, planned, one to one, professional supervision from registered and appropriately experienced social workers.	Managers should arrange appropriate professional supervision for social workers, particularly in multidisciplinary teams or specialist roles. Social workers need to take responsibility for ensuring they have access to and use professional supervision and discussion.
CASW	No national policy. Under provincial/ territorial authorities. Social workers strive to facilitate access to appropriate professional consultation or supervision for professional social work practice.	Social workers have a responsibility to maintain professional proficiency, to continually strive to increase their professional knowledge and skills . . . seeking consultation and supervision as appropriate. CASW (Code of Ethics)
Hong Kong SWRB	Recent graduates have an especially strong need for supervision in order to consolidate the knowledge and skills acquired during their studies, to successfully manage the stress that accompanies their new responsibilities, and to be adequately prepared to become supervisors themselves.	Social workers with three or more years of full-time experience should have the equivalent of one uninterrupted hour of supervision in every two months. If supervision is conducted by a peer (a colleague of the same rank), the responsibility for accountability and review should be assumed by someone in a senior position.
IASW	All professionally qualified social work delivered supervision is accrued at the rate of one point per hour of supervision. It is necessary to gain a minimum number of 20 points in the supervision category but no maximum number of points is set. Supervision Minimum 20 points per 2 year CPD cycle required for Full Time Social Workers (10 CPD points for part time Social Workers).	CPD: While the IASW preference is for all social workers to have individual supervision from their line managers, the IASW are aware that this is not possible for all social workers at present, so the IASW will accept social work consultation. IASW will also accept up to 25% or 5 of the 20 CPD points required via group supervision facilitated by a suitably trained social work line manager or senior social worker.
South Africa	Supervision of all social workers is mandatory. Only social workers may act as social workers' supervisors. SA Social Service Professions Act (110 of 1978) and specifically according to the Code of Ethics, which is part of the Act (also attached – see specifically point 5.4.1 of the Code).	Social workers do not get CPD points for supervision as supervision is mandatory. . . . Supervision services may be outsourced. The supervision of social workers may thus be conducted by a social worker not in the employment of the organisation and may be obtained on a contractual basis as "external supervision".

(continued)

Table 1 continued

Professional body/regulator	Supervision requirements	Links to licensing and ongoing professional development
Singapore Association of Social Workers	To be registered requires obtaining a recognised social work degree or graduate diploma and have 1,000 supervised practice hours from a qualified supervisor before, during and/ or after their studies. The supervision may be conducted on an individual or group basis.	CPD: Receiving supervision from a supervisor with a recognised social work degree and at least 3 years of social work experience. The total number of supervision hours should not exceed four hours per month or for group, eight hours per month.

Sources: Aotearoa New Zealand Association of Social Workers (ANZASW), and the Social Workers Registration Board in New Zealand (SWRB), the Australian Association of Social Workers (AASW), the British Association of Social Workers (BASW), the Association of Social Work Boards (ASWB), the Irish Association of Social Workers (IASW), the Canadian Association of Social Workers (CASW), National Association of Social Workers (NASW), Social Workers Registration Board Hong Kong, and South African Council for Social Service Professions (SACSSP) (and additional information provided via Engelbrecht, 2014, personal communication).

In a more recent study Hair (2013) found that one quarter of her participants felt that developmental supervision for knowledge and skill development needed to be time-limited for up to three years. Continuing supervision was seen to challenge social worker "professional autonomy, work credibility and potentially the respect of other professionals", and one of Hair's participants stated that "supervision must have an end point just like childhood" (2013, p. 1577). "Perpetual" supervision would need to be replaced by consultation–conversations between social workers or between social workers and senior clinicians from other disciplines. While this concern has not been subject to recent study elsewhere it seems possible that acceptance of a traditional approach to supervision should not be assumed to be universal.

Whether or not social workers continue to participate in supervision throughout their careers, they will experience changes in their skills and competence, and will require support and encouragement for professional development. While consultation, group-based peer support and interprofessional supervision may be explored as alternatives to traditional one–to-one "line management" supervision, it can be seen from Table 1 that the latter has a firm hold on the profession. Egan's study of Australian social workers found that nearly two-thirds of respondents identified their supervisor as internal to their team and two-thirds were also line managers; 22.3% had supervisors external to their team; and 81.6% of respondents did not have a choice of supervisor (Egan, 2012, p. 177). This in spite of the critique of supervision described above, and the impact of greater managerial control of social work (Noble & Irwin, 2009) demonstrate that social work is hanging on tightly to a traditional model. Rather than weakening the profession's control, the risk averse and surveillant managerialism in social work organisations has paradoxically strengthened supervision (Beddoe, 2011). It is in the early career that there is a fairly strong consensus that supervision is of great value.

Early Career Practitioners

Early career social workers are characterised often as "green" as in new, untested and a mix of uncertainty and enthusiasm (Franklin, 2011). Supervision in the social work placement will have inducted the novice social worker into the world of professional practitioners and much of their understanding of practice will have been experienced through interaction with experienced practitioners and service users, the latter often carefully monitored and observed. Good placements will have provided the opportunity to test out students' capacity to demonstrate critical thinking. Sensitive supervision will have provided a safe place for students to be guided toward safe use of self: a "reflective process minimises blame, shame and doubt and identifies and applies creative and individual strategies in self-care and professional development to further strengthen their practice" (Marlowe, Appleton & Chinnery, 2014, p. 11). However, most social workers will agree that placement is not "the real thing" and the early years are exciting but can be very demanding. In an ideal world all would have access to a structured early career programme such as the English model reported by Carpenter, Patsios et al. (2013). This programme included dedicated time for professional development and supervision of the beginning practitioners, supporting materials for participants and supporting materials and comprehensive training for supervisors and programme coordinators.

Given the considerable investment made in pre-service education for social work (by students, academics, practice educators and other stakeholders) little is done in many countries to support the needs of newly qualified practitioners, beyond an induction programme which may be offered by some larger employing agencies. For those beginning work in smaller organisations their support needs will be met by colleagues and their supervisor. Access to further professional development may be limited and continuing professional education is frequently only available for those willing to self-fund and use personal leave. The latter situation in the author's own country means that practitioners' hopes that greater regulation of social work would lead to better resourcing for further professional development has not been borne out (Beddoe, 2013). For early career social workers however supervision has benefited from mandatory requirements set by regulators. As shown in Table 1 earlier in this chapter licensing or full registration often requires adherence to minimum hours of supervision in the period following qualification, thus ensuring (at least in theory) that supervision must be made available. Research shows that this doesn't always mean that there is full compliance with expectations as in several jurisdictions practitioners were not receiving regular supervision (Baginsky et al., 2010; Egan, 2012; Robinson, 2013). In England recent research has examined the provision of supervision for beginning practitioners. Manthorpe, Moriarty, Hussein, Stevens and Sharpe (2013) sought the views of newly qualified social workers, managers and directors on various elements of their support and development in their jobs. Among the findings was that those who had less frequent supervision were less likely to feel they had a manageable workload and to be less engaged with the job. They also found links that may suggest that the informal supervision provided by supportive team members may be more effective than traditional line management supervision. Space does not allow for a more detailed exploration of the needs of early career practitioners but it seems clear that high quality supervision, structured and informal team/peer support is vital and needs resources for development and evaluation. Social work supervision provided by an experienced social worker is most appropriate at this stage.

Mature Practitioners: Holding the Line and Holding on to Hopefulness

Supervision in social work does continue as practitioners shift from beginners to mature and seasoned practitioners and seems to be valued. Research by Hair (2013, p. 1577) reported that 80 percent of respondents in a Canadian study believed that that supervision did not need to end and despite the doubts of some noted earlier in this chapter, 78 percent were clear that career long supervision was not associated with "reduced professional autonomy". In Hair's (2013) study, advocates of career-long supervision did agree that supervision would change over time, and as noted earlier supervision should depart form a "power over" model of supervision and evolve to a more consultative model. Those who supported enduring supervision found it essential for continuing accountability and development. Hair (2013, p. 1577) notes that the strongest reason for career long supervision was for emotional support (77 percent), followed closely by the need for professional development (75 percent). Thus supervision is closely tied to both professional development and the long term need for emotional support in social work. Social work is characterised as demanding and can be corrosive to wellbeing. Indeed the literature abounds with a theme of the dangers of social work for resilience and wellbeing and employers have naturally focussed on supervision as a support for staff retention. Research has provided ample evidence of the links between practitioner support and wellbeing and retention in different countries and different fields of practice (McFadden, Campbell & Taylor, 2014; Shier & Graham, 2011; Ellett, Ellis, Westbrook & Dews, 2007; Pockett, 2002). Astvik, Melin and Allvin (2013, p. 52) in Sweden have identified five different main types of strategies: "compensatory, demand-reducing, disengagement, voice and exit". Compensatory strategies ("the mobilisation of compensatory effort to deal with the imbalance between work demands and available resources") were used by nearly all their participants in order to maintain levels of performance (Astvik et al., p. 56). The strategies included overtime, taking work home, skipping breaks and working while sick, and the extensive use of such strategies was connected with negative outcomes in health.

In recent years there has been some shift towards trying to focus on the positive factors which might influence practitioners' decisions to stay in their jobs and what helps people thrive rather than just survive (Collins, 2007; Wendt, Tuckey & Prosser, 2011). Studies have previously noted that, even when emotional exhaustion in social work is high, certain organisational features and personal characteristics may allow workers to remain satisfied with their jobs (Wendt et al., 2001; Mandell, Stalker, de Zeeuw Wright, Frensch & Harvey, 2013). Such features include organisational, supervisory, team and peer support as noted by Baines et al. (2014) in non-government organisations, by Mandell et al. (2013) in child welfare, and in health practice (Beddoe,

Davys & Adamson, 2014). Individual characteristics such as "personal commitment to the mission" of social work, strong values, and a personality that is supportive and sensitive to the needs of others are also significant (Mandell et al., 2013, p. 384). Wendt et al. (2011) have emphasised the importance of the personal domain, where beliefs, values, and personal/professional boundaries are highly sustaining. A recent qualitative study by Pooler, Wolfer and Freeman (2014) utilised an appreciative inquiry approach to explore social workers who found joy in their work. Participants identified interpersonal factors of making connections and making a difference and intrapersonal (making meaning and making a life) sources of joy and "reflected significant personal initiative in the process of finding joy" (p. 1).

So what are the implications for supervision? Supervision continues to play a part in social work over the career span and clearly has a role to play in mediating the challenges and stresses of the job and in supporting practitioners to hold on to a positive, hopeful focus on "the mission" and values. Given there may be some tension around the traditional hierarchical model of supervision for those "staying put" in social work it is useful to consider other forms of supervision.

Modes of Supervision

While one-to-one supervision is evidently still the norm in social work in many countries, other approaches have been developed and further research is needed to evaluate their impact, especially on the needs of mature practitioners. Group and peer options and interprofessional supervision are increasingly used, sometime for pragmatic reasons – efficiency, providing supervision to those separated by rural and remote locations – and sometimes to bring more knowledge and perspectives into the supervision process. In this section group and peer supervision will be briefly explored and the challenges of supervision between people from different professions – interprofessional supervision – will be examined.

Group and Peer Supervision

For mature practitioners group supervision may be considered useful to augment or even replace one-to-one supervision. Group supervision can be a supplement to the individual meeting and is often recommended as an efficient use of time and as a vehicle where social workers can learn from each other. The group or peer mode of supervision offers an experience of sharing common challenges and can additionally "normalize reactions to stressful work environments and practice experiences, and alleviate isolation" (Bogo & McKnight, 2006, p. 53). Self-identified resilient practitioners in one study emphasised the importance of peer support in maintaining hopeful practice (Beddoe et al., 2014). Peer group supervision offers much more than just a more cost effective mode of supervision delivery–with attention to good process and the absence of a supervisor in an authority role, power and control issues are diminished, and a "mutual aid model can flourish" (Bogo & McKnight, 2006, p. 53).

There is also ongoing interest in the importance of informal or ad hoc peer support and supervision which may happen quite spontaneously and yet is noted frequently as significant in providing non-hierarchical sharing of ideas and experience both in field education amongst students and practitioners and in practice between qualified colleagues (Golia & McGovern, 2013). Learning to effectively and appropriately seek support, collegial advice and task assistance are important professional qualities in social work and provision of opportunities to do this in groups whether facilitated or informal are undoubtedly useful to augment supervision.

Interprofessional Supervision

Hair (2013, p. 1567) cites Tsui (2005, p. 37) in noting that in general the social work supervision literature appears to assume that "both supervisor and supervisee are professional social workers" who hold in common the values, norms and aims of social work and its ethical standards. That this is not universal is indicated by the emergence of cross-disciplinary supervision, now most frequently referred to as interprofessional supervision (IPS) a new phenomenon. There are several possible explanations for this development; one of the most likely is the intensification in demands for supervision where organisations and professional bodies set expectations. It is not known if there is an international shortage of supervisors but Egan (2012) has noted in Australia that workforce dynamics and lack of education and training opportunities for current and potential supervisors may coalesce to create strain on supervisory capacity. The other factor that has influenced the development of interprofessional supervision is found perhaps more in adult social work. Berger and Mizrahi (2001) and Bogo, Paterson, Tufford and King (2011) have noted that over the last few decades many unitary social work departments have disappeared, replaced with the embedding of social workers and other allied health professionals within amalgamated services. Berger and Mizrahi (2001, p. 5) noted that practice groups were "decentralized, combining disciplines and resources under a single, unifying structure, led by a generic manager". In a survey of 750 hospitals in the USA it was found that cross-disciplinary arrangements had increased, raising questions about supervisory philosophy and method and potentially weakened understanding of professional education, scope of practice and roles within such interdisciplinary teams (Berger & Mizrahi, 2001). The focus on interprofessional collaboration and education within health services in particular has also contributed to some dilution of traditional expectations of same-profession supervision.

Over the past decade several researchers have expressed concerns about the growth of interprofessional supervision without specific training or mandate being required (see for example, in counselling: Crocket et al., 2009; and in social work: O'Donoghue, 2004). While it seems likely that mandates and professional regulation may limit the growth of interprofessional supervision, it is now a feature of the mosaic of supervision arrangements for social work, and so some exploration is warranted.

Strong et al. (2004) asked about interprofessional supervision in a study of supervision practice in allied health professions in an Australian setting. While there were divergent views they found a consensus on three important concerns: that IPS might result in "the devaluing of the specific skills of the disciplines" (psychology, occupational therapy, speech pathology, and social work); that a "clash in frameworks" might lead to "guidance, modelling, and direction" in clinical matters being inappropriate, and that IPS might provide a vehicle for the implementation of a generic mental health worker model which was the source of alarm amongst the professional groups (Strong et al., 2004, p. 202). The greatest concern was for new graduates, who were thought to be more vulnerable in IPS "to the loss of professional identity associated with the oversimplification of discipline skills" (p. 202.). The research of Strong et al. also noted some benefits of IPS provided "ground rules were observed such as supervisee choice and continuing access to discipline specific supervision", with one of their participants noting that IPS could "provide new ideas, new grasp of things if there is basic trust, but it needs to be a two-way street" (Strong et al., 2004, pp. 202–3).

Exploration of the potential benefits of supervision between different professionals finds a consistent agreement about the need for collaboration and cooperation between professions with the potential to improve teamwork and interprofessionality (Townend, 2005; Chipchase, Allen, Eley, McAllister & Strong, 2012). The term "interprofessional" itself reflects the assumption that collaboration among professionals will lead to improved care for service users (Bogo et al., 2011). The interprofessional agenda poses a reconciliation of professional differences through education and shared decision making. And thus within this framework, supervision would be congruent with an emphasis on the integration of approaches where the participants share knowledge to come up with new or refined multidisciplinary approaches to work with service users. Several studies have explored interprofessional arrangements. Townend (2005) found interprofessional supervision was instrumental in bringing together skills; sharing information; enhancing continuity of care; clarifying responsibilities and accountabilities; planning resources; and delivering expert resources in counselling and psychotherapy services. Bogo et al. (2011, p. 133) found ambivalence amongst mental health practitioners but general agreement emerged that the key characteristics of valued supervisors include their clinical expertise and the "ability to provide new and relevant practice knowledge in a respectful and safe process". In a study of nurses in mental health Mullarkey, Keeley & Playle (2001) reported that enhanced learning from an interprofessional supervision improves understanding of the specific contributions of different professional groups to client care.

More recently Beddoe and Howard (2012) undertook a study of interprofessional supervision with two professional groups in New Zealand, social workers and psychologists. All respondents were either in receipt of interprofessional supervision or providing it. Of the 243 respondents 28.2% were psychologists and 71.8% were social workers. In an online survey respondents were asked about the perceived benefits and disadvantages of receiving interprofessional supervision. Beddoe and Howard reported most frequently cited benefits of receiving IPS by supervisees were the "usefulness of different approaches/perspectives"; "increases my knowledge"; "facilitates creative thinking"; "more creative outcomes"; "enhances my understanding of other professional approaches"; "helps me question my institutional approach" (2012, p. 187). Survey respondents were also asked about the circumstances in which they believed interprofessional supervision worked effectively. Themes reported by Beddoe and Howard confirmed earlier literature in "recognising the advantages of a fresh perspective, specialist knowledge and skills gained in an IPS relationship" (p. 187). Circumstances favouring effective interprofessional supervision included: knowledge gaps being better met by another discipline with specialist expertise; consultation on specific and difficult cases, where new research findings might be addressed; in order to support cultural perspectives and needs; and creating distance from workplace dynamics (pp. 187–188). Echoing support for external supervision (Bradley & Höjer, 2009; Beddoe, 2011) the IPS study noted the search for supervision in a neutral space, one respondent writing:

> There is no contamination from interpersonal office politics and dynamics at times when supervision [needs to be] a place to look at those issues and re-think strategies. (Beddoe & Howard, 2012, p. 188)

This perceived neutral space fostered greater openness, an "outsider" view beyond the dynamics of team and organisational, and released from the potential tensions of hierarchical relationships.

The disadvantages reported in relation to interprofessional supervision are often linked to potential conflicts or competitive relations between professional groups. It is often argued that only highly experienced practitioners should embark on an interdisciplinary relationship; at a stage where professional identity is relatively well-defined and there are clear and compatible learning needs. Chipchase et al. (2012) studied interprofessional supervision in pre-service clinical training and found that students had varied views about such arrangements, many stating that they wanted their same-profession supervisor available throughout clinical placements. Participants in a study by Bogo et al. (2011, p. 132) recommended different supervision arrangements be available at different stages in clinicians' careers and for new inexperienced clinicians, profession-specific supervision is deemed more appropriate. Beddoe and Howard (2012) found the most frequently stated disadvantages of IPS by supervisees were "aspects of my professional role are not adequately addressed"; "not all issues can be raised with the supervisor"; "lack of shared theories or language"; "disempowerment due to professional status differences"; and "my supervisor is not familiar with the ethical standards of my profession" (Beddoe & Howard, 2012, p. 189). Thus supervisors were very cognisant of professional difference in codes, theoretical bases and some noted that there was a need to manage carefully the risk of one perspective dominating supervision: "I have to watch carefully if my psych perspective dominates, and temper it" and a social worker noted he/she had to be careful not to "colonize the supervisee with a social justice way of being" (Beddoe & Howard, 2012, p. 190). These reports suggest that it is timely to consider how supervisors are trained for their potential role in IPS (Davys & Beddoe, 2008).

Conclusions

A chapter such as this can only begin to gather together the themes which emerge when we consider the supervisor needs of supervisees across the career span. There are remaining questions regarding what modes might work best and the implications for supervisor training. This chapter has not addressed "what works" for the development of supervisors, an area ripe for further investigation. In particular if interprofessional supervision is to become more popular at mid and later career stages, how best do we prepare supervisors and supervisees to make the most of this mode? Given the importance placed on supervision within our profession it is vital that such research and development continues.

References

Aotearoa New Zealand Association of Social Workers (2012). *Supervision Policy*. Christchurch: ANZASW.

Association of Social Work Boards (2009). *An Analysis of Supervision for Social Work Licensure: Guidelines on supervision for regulators and educators*. Culpeper VA: Author. Retrieved from http://www.aswb.org/wpcontent/uploads/2013/10/supervisionjobanalysis.pdf

Association of Social Work Boards (ASWB) (2006–12). Social Work Licensing FAQs: Licensing and Social Work Boards: What kind of supervision should I be getting? Retrieved at http://www.aswb.org/faqs/what-kind-of-supervision-should-i-be-getting/

Astvik, W., Melin, M., & Allvin, M. (2013). Survival strategies in social work: A study of how coping strategies affect service quality, professionalism and employee health. *Nordic Social Work Research, 4*(1), 52–66.

Australian Association of Social Workers (2014). *AASW Supervision Standards*. Canberra: Australian Association of Social Workers. Retrieved from http://www.aasw.asn.au/practitioner-resources/ethics-standards

Baginsky, M., Moriarty, J., Manthorpe, J., Stevens, M., MacInnes, T., & Nagendran, T. (2010). Social workers' workload survey messages from the frontline: Findings from the 2009 survey and interviews with senior managers. Leeds, Children's Workforce Development Council, and King's College London.

Baines, D., Charlesworth, S., Turner, D., & O'Neill, L. (2014). Lean social care and worker identity: The role of outcomes, supervision and mission. *Critical Social Policy*. doi:10.1177/0261018314538799

Beddoe, L. (2011). External supervision in social work: Power, space, risk, and the search for safety. *Australian Social Work, 65*(2), 197–213. doi:10.1080/0312407x.2011.591187

Beddoe, L. (2013). Continuing education, registration and professional identity in New Zealand social work. *International Social Work*. doi:10.1177/0020872812473139

Beddoe, L., Davys, A. M., & Adamson, C. (2014). 'Never trust anybody who says "I don't need supervision"': Practitioners' beliefs about social worker resilience. *Practice, 26*(2), 113–130. doi:10.1080/09503153.2014.896888

Beddoe, L., & Howard, F. (2012). Interprofessional supervision in social work and psychology: Mandates and (inter) professional relationships. *The Clinical Supervisor, 31*(2), 178–202. doi:10.1080/07325223.2013.730471

Berger, C., & Mizrahi, T. (2001). An evolving paradigm of supervision within a changing health care environment. *Social Work in Health Care, 32*(4), 1–18.

Bogo, M., & McKnight, K. (2006). 'Clinical supervision in social work: A review of the research literature'. *The Clinical Supervisor, 24*(1/2), 49–67.

Bogo, M., Paterson, J., Tufford, L., & King, R. (2011). Interprofessional clinical supervision in mental health and addiction: Toward identifying common elements. *The Clinical Supervisor, 30*(1), 124–140.

Bradley, G., & Höjer, S. (2009). Supervision reviewed: Reflections on two different social work models in England and Sweden. *European Journal of Social Work, 12*(1), 71–85.

British Association of Social Workers (2011). *Supervision Policy*. UK: Ethics, and Human Rights Committee, the British Association of Social Workers. Retrieved from http://cdn.basw.co.uk/upload/basw_73346–6.pdf

Carpenter, J., Webb, C. M., & Bostock, L. (2013). The surprisingly weak evidence base for supervision: Findings from a systematic review of research in child welfare practice (2000–2012). *Children and Youth Services Review, 35*(11), 1843–1853. doi:http://dx.doi.org/10.1016/j.childyouth.2013.08.014

Carpenter, J., Patsios, D., Wood, M., Platt, D., Shardlow, S., Mclaughlin, H., Blewett, J. (2013). Early Professional Development Pilot Programme (First cohort 2009 to 2011): Final Evaluation Report. London: Department for Education.

Chipchase, L., Allen, S., Eley, D., McAllister, L., & Strong, J. (2012). Interprofessional supervision in an intercultural context: A qualitative study. *Journal of Interprofessional Care, 26*(6), 465–471. doi:10.3109/13561820.2012.718813

Collins, S. (2007). Social workers, resilience, positive emotions and optimism. *Practice, 19*(4), 255–269.

Crocket, K., Cahill, F., Flanagan, P., Franklin, J., McGill, R., Stewart, A., Mulcahy, D. (2009). Possibilities and limits of cross-disciplinary supervision. *New Zealand Journal of Counselling, 29*(2), 25–43.

Davys, A., & Beddoe, L. (2008). Interprofessional learning for supervision: 'Taking the blinkers off'. *Learning in Health and Social Care, 8*(1), 58–69. doi: 10.1111/j.1473–6861.2008.00197.x

Egan, R. (2012). Australian social work supervision practice in 2007. *Australian Social Work, 65*(2), 171–184. doi:10.1080/0312407x.2011.653575

Ellett, A. J., Ellis, J. I., Westbrook, T. M., & Dews, D. (2007). A qualitative study of 369 child welfare professionals' perspectives about factors contributing to employee retention and turnover. *Children and Youth Services Review, 29*(2), 264–281.

Franklin, L. D. (2011). Reflective supervision for the green social worker: Practical applications for supervisors. *The Clinical Supervisor, 30*(2), 204–214. doi:10.1080/07325223.2011.607743

Golia, G. M., & McGovern, A. R. (2013). If you save me, I'll save you: The power of peer supervision in clinical training and professional development. *British Journal of Social Work*. doi:10.1093/bjsw/bct138

Hair, H. J. (2013). The purpose and duration of supervision, and the training and discipline of supervisors: What social workers say they need to provide effective services. *British Journal of Social Work, 43*(8), 1562–1588. doi:10.1093/bjsw/bcs071

Irish Association of Social Workers (2009). *Continuing Professional Development Policy*. Retrieved from: https://www.iasw.ie/attachments/07071812-cfe6–4604-a86a-cbbdb37a76f0.PDF

Laufer, H. (2004). Long-experienced social workers and supervision: Perceptions and implications, *The Clinical Supervisor, 22*(2), pp. 153–71.

Mandell, D., Stalker, C., de Zeeuw Wright, M., Frensch, K., & Harvey, C. (2013). Sinking, swimming and sailing: Experiences of job satisfaction and emotional exhaustion in child welfare employees. *Child & Family Social Work, 18*(4), 383–393.

Manthorpe, J., Moriarty, J., Hussein, S., Stevens, M., & Sharpe, E. (2013). Content and purpose of supervision in social work practice in England: Views of newly qualified social workers, managers and directors. *British Journal of Social Work*. doi:10.1093/bjsw/bct102

Marlowe, J. M., Appleton, C., Chinnery, S.-A., & Van Stratum, S. (2014). The integration of personal and professional selves: Developing students' critical awareness in social work practice. *Social Work Education, 34*(1), 1–14. doi:10.1080/02615479.2014.949230

McFadden, P., Campbell, A., & Taylor, B. (2014). Resilience and burnout in child protection social work: Individual and organisational themes from a systematic literature review. *British Journal of Social Work*. doi:10.1093/bjsw/bct210

Mullarkey, K., Keeley, P., & Playle, J. F. (2001). Multiprofessional clinical supervision: Challenges for mental health nurses. *Journal of Psychiatric and Mental Health Nursing, 8*(3), 205–211. DOI: 10.1046/j.1365–2850.2001.00376.x

National Association of Social Workers (NASW) (2005). *NASW Standards for Clinical Social Work in Social Work Practice*. Washington, DC: Author.

Noble, C., & Irwin, J. (2009). Social work supervision: An exploration of the current challenges in a rapidly changing social, economic and political environment. *Journal of Social Work, 9*(3), 345–358. doi:10.1177/1468017309334848

O'Donoghue, K. (2004). Social workers and cross-disciplinary supervision. *Social Work Review, 16*(3), 2–7.

Pockett, R. (2002). Staying in hospital social work. *Social Work in Health Care, 36*(3), 1–24. doi:10.1300/J010v36n03_01

Pooler, D., Wolfer, T., & Freeman, M. (2014). Finding joy in social work: Interpersonal sources. *Families in Society*. doi:10.1606/1044–3894.2014.95.5

Robinson, K. (2013). Supervision found wanting: Experiences of health and social workers in non-government organisations working with refugees and asylum seekers. *Practice, 25*(2), 87–103. doi:10.1080/09503153.2013.775238

Shier, M. L., & Graham, J. R. (2011). Work-related factors that impact social work practitioners' subjective well-being: Well-being in the workplace. *Journal of Social Work, 11*(4), 402–421.

Social Workers Registration Board (New Zealand) (2013). *Supervision Expectations for Registered Social Workers: Policy Statement*. Wellington: SWRB. Retrieved from swrb.govt.nz/policy

Social Workers Registration Board (Hong Kong) (2009). Guidelines for Social Work Supervision. Retrieved from http://www.swrb.org.hk/engasp/supervision_c.asp

South African Council for Social Service Professions (2007). Policy guidelines for course of conduct, code of ethics and the rules for social workers. SACSSP. Available at http://www.sacssp.co.za/website/wp-content/uploads/ 2012/06/Code-of-Ethics.pdf

Strong, J., Kavanagh, D., Wilson, J., Spence, S. H., Worrall, L., & Crow, N. (2004). Supervision practice for allied health professionals within a large mental health service. *The Clinical Supervisor, 22*(1), 191–210.

Tsui, M.-s. (2005). *Social work supervision: Contexts and concepts*. Thousand Oaks: Sage.

Veeder, N. W. (1991). Autonomy, accountability, and professionalism: The case against close supervision in social work. *The Clinical Supervisor, 8*(2), 33–47.

Wendt, S., Tuckey, M. R., & Prosser, B. (2011). Thriving, not just surviving, in emotionally demanding fields of practice. *Health & Social Care in the Community, 19*(3), 317–325.

Wonnacott, J. (2013). *Supervision: a luxury or critical to good practice in times of austerity*. Paper presented at the Bournemouth University National Centre for Post Qualifying Social Work Conference: Child Protection in a Time of Austerity, Bournemouth. http://www.in-trac.co.uk/news/supervision-in-times-of-austerity/ 6a03c7acce6&groupId=10180

Using Visual Cues to Develop a Practice Framework in Student Supervision

Jane Maidment

School of Language, Social and Political Sciences, University of Canterbury, Christchurch, New Zealand

Abstract

This chapter discusses ways to develop a practice framework as part of student supervision process. In particular, methods to incorporate the use of visual learning strategies to develop the practice framework are examined. The educational scaffolding for developing a framework is outlined and processes for helping students to create their own are identified. Use of visual aids such as brainstorming and metaphor, as part of the design for the framework are examined. Brainstorming and metaphor have proven to be useful devices to enhance meaningful engagement and ownership of ideas for the visual learner (Willox, Harper, Bridger, Orbach & Sarapura, 2010; Edwards & Cooper, 2010). Fostering peer generated critical reflection, reflexivity, and critical thinking within and outside of placement supervision generates a constructivist learning environment, enabling students to draw the threads of their own framework together through dialogue with others. Throughout the chapter, the conceptual ideas discussed are illustrated using personal narratives from a former student and a current student supervisor who both prepared a practice framework as part of their own professional development.

Introduction

Providing supervision to students is one of the most formative tasks that can be undertaken in educating for future social work practice. The role of the supervisor is integral in helping students develop a professional identity, forge an understanding of how theory and practice integrate and assist in the cultivation of a personal practitioner style. Developing a practice framework as part of student placement supervision adds strength to integrating theory, practice, personal values and policy knowledge. As such the supervisor is a powerful influence in terms of mentoring, supporting and challenging students at the beginning of their social work career, while encouraging significant professional socialisation. Within the process of delivering supervision it is important to understand that students engage in learning via diverse pathways. This diversity signals the need to use a variety of teaching and learning techniques within supervision to foster rich and in-depth student learning while on placement. This chapter focuses on how visual prompts and processes can be used to enhance student supervision. To illustrate the application of theory and the impact of creating practice frameworks, narratives from Liam (a former student) and Cathie (a student supervisor) are incorporated into this chapter. Both Liam and Cathie have created their own practice frameworks and continue to use them to inform their social work and supervision.

Putting the "Visual" into Supervision Learning

One of the most well-known typologies of experiential learning styles that readily relates to the social work practicum was developed by David Kolb. Kolb differentiated between students who preferred to engage in learning via concrete experience, active experimentation, reflective observation, or abstract conceptualisation (1984). Further distinctions have been made between student preferences for visual and verbal learning strategies (Mayer & Massa, 2003; Felder & Soloman, 2004), which also readily transpose into the context of student supervision in social work. Having an understanding of the student learning style enables supervision to be performed in ways that enable information, skill and knowledge acquisition to occur, be retained and enjoyed, using the most effective means. Much student supervision in social work is carried out using verbal techniques alone, mirroring "talk therapies" that inevitably privilege auditory learners. However, an American study of university students has revealed that approximately 40% are visual learners, preferring to be taught by integrating pictures, film, diagrams, flow charts and demonstrations into the instruction (Clarke, Flaherty & Yankey, 2006). More specifically in social work education, very little has been published about use of images and visual interpretation for theorising, practice or learning (Huss, 2012). Despite this paucity of information frequent use of visual aids occurs in work with service users who do not readily engage with complex issues in word based forms, such as children, people with intellectual disabilities (Walton, 2012) or those who have had a stroke. Both Cathie and Liam noted how visual cues strengthened their engagement in education and with clients.

Liam commented . . .

> My wall mounted year planner played a prominent role during my studies. I used it as a tool for reminding me of due dates for assignments. During class time we used to complete exercises in groups where we would write our responses to questions on butcher's papers. I used to find this really useful to look at when other groups would present back to class. Otherwise I can't really remember other visual tools like that of the framework. It would have been great to have developed something like it in Year 1 and changed and modified it during the degree.

Things visual are also important to Cathie who noted. . .

> I use visual heaps. I scribble things when talking to clients; I have sayings on the wall that I change regularly, likewise posters. I also change posters at the front occasionally, so clients aren't seeing the 'same old, same old' every time they come in. I'm a hopeless artist but I don't let that stop me – as long as the client/student/supervisee gets it, that's the point.

Utilising the visual techniques of brainstorming together with metaphor as vehicles for developing a practice framework, are suggested in the guidelines below. The purpose of generating these visual representations is to enable the relationships between parts of a "whole" to be illustrated. The process of developing a practice framework via visual modalities enables students to see and articulate the "big picture" while showing the linkages between the essential components. Using visual cues in this way enhances both student understanding and memory retention of content (Higgins, 1994). Additional advantages of using visual methodologies for learning include the possibility for opening up new and empowering narratives and different ways of thinking; the therapeutic quality of image making is in itself a "health" activity; use of colour, shape and contours add semantic and emotional detail; with image enabling the articulation of different forms of social experience that are hard to express through language, text and numbers alone (Huss, 2012, pp. 1442–1443). Visual representation also facilitates students incorporating their own choice of content, medium and product; involves the assemblage and presentation of subtle thinking, feeling, action and context in professional encounters; is able to incorporate one or more of multiple mediums including craft, multimedia design or art in two or three dimensional forms; is not constrained by the imposition of chronology as the major organising factor (Walton, 2012). In summary Marshall (2007, p. 3) argues that forms of art making allows "information to be seen differently, in a fresh, more meaningful, personal and experiential way (as in art, symbolism and metaphor). This transformation of concepts through imaging produces new insights and learning".

Research into using visual processing as opposed to predominately verbal discussion in counsellor supervision found drawing methods were more effective than verbal processing when analysing for student understanding of crisis counselling (Stone & Admundson, 1989 cited in Deaver & Shiflett, 2011, p. 261) Further, using visual strategies within the context of supervision and practice journaling result in generating increased self-awareness and greater understanding of client issues (Deaver & McAuliffe, 2009; Guiffrida, Jordan, Saiz & Barnes, 2007).

As part of supervision in social work field education students routinely write up workbooks, portfolios and reflective journals. Within the context of completing these largely text-based documents to demonstrate placement learning, supervisors can encourage use of visual representation. Images might be used to demonstrate such things as seating arrangements in a family or team gathering as well as depicting the atmosphere of the meeting; expression of ambivalence about an ethical dilemma and the contributing factors; demonstration of emotion about an intervention outcome; or creation of a visual typology of a practice journey with a client, group or community. Such images can be used to explore the dynamics of the incidents themselves and tease out the resultant student learning during supervision. Together, the development of a visual representation of theory/practice linkages alongside use of metaphor provides a powerful means of expressing a fully integrated practice framework.

Use of Metaphor

The construction of a metaphor is "an analytical device that assist with understanding of an unknown situation in terms of a familiar one" (Lakoff, 1993 cited in Coleman, Rourke & Allen, 2012, p. 136). Common metaphors of speech include, "Love is a journey",

"Flogging a dead horse" and "Don't judge a book by its cover". Developing the practice framework using a graphic metaphor enables students to connect their conceptual knowledge with a visual image, scene or experience that is significant to them. Common pictorial metaphors seen in art include the bridge, the garden, the road and the mountain.

A great deal has been written about ways in which using metaphor can generate deep learning for students in higher education, noting in particular that metaphors foster meaning making out of conceptual and abstract content; generate new ideas and reframe understanding; help define the "intangible or abstract"; increase retention of knowledge and allows for potentially unfamiliar ideas to be connected with the familiar (Willox et al., 2010, p. 71).

Liam explains how he decided upon what metaphor to use for his practice framework . . .

> I had just purchased a new manual for my Mini. In the manual was an early 60's promotional image of a side on mini cut in half from front to back. I remember looking at all the different components that made up the mini. I thought, and still do, that it is a unique and well-designed car. The amount of time that had been taken to make sure that every element worked in harmony with the other was clearly visible in the image. It was at this point that I suddenly made the connection to practice. Once I had a go at scribbling some social work concepts to the image it just started to make sense and I began to build and run with the idea from that point.

Duffy, writing about use of metaphor in social work practice, explains that metaphors enable clients (or in this case students) to discover dimensions of reality and meaning not previously considered; by-pass resistant postures; create a verbal play space; highlight the moment; promote interaction around a shared image; allow for explorations that are culturally meaningful; and link the imaginative and the cognitive functioning (Gans, 1991 cited in Duffy, 2005, p. 254).

These elements are evident in Liam's description of how he chose the "Mini" as a metaphor above, and in Cathie's choice of metaphor. . .

> I started with an umbrella. But the imagery wasn't working for me and then I was talking about a "toolbox" with someone, I thought that might be a useful metaphor. The kete [woven flax bag] was a natural follow on and I like so many things about it – particularly the idea that it's woven and that in being woven, it gains strength and usefulness. Also, it can hold a variety of tools. I've got a sort of crossword effect on it as well, with the various components that I use. The interwoven-ness of how I practice is important to me, so that's what I use.

Cathie used the metaphor of a kete (flax woven basket made by Maori) to develop her practice framework.

Duffy goes on to explain "The metaphor is one of the most basic mechanisms for understanding our experiences. When we construct metaphors, we use both sides of the brain, the intuitive and the rational, with the potential of generating new understanding, new realities, and new behaviours" (Duffy, 2005, p. 247). After describing current contemporary social work education specifically in the area of human development as "anaemic", Forte advocates for use of the metaphor in teaching as a way of

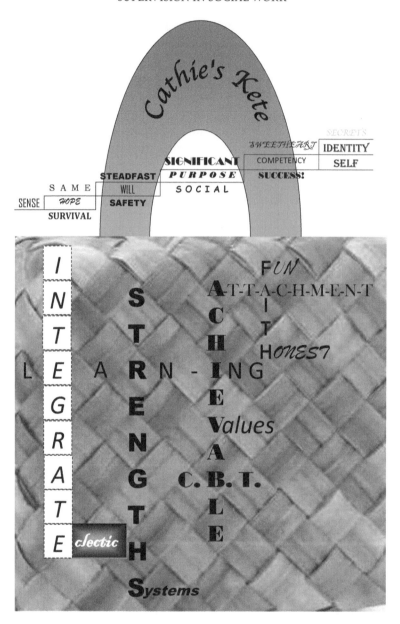

including the "imaginative and educational use of comparisons between theoretical ideas and everyday events, objects, processes, people and places" (Forte, 2009, p. 943). As such, the device of metaphor appears to be well suited for use in developing the practice framework, straddling as it does the spheres of theoretical consciousness and the seemingly mundane awareness of everyday living.

Liam explains how he worked with his metaphor to begin conceptualising important components of practice. . .

The process was surprisingly easy once the metaphor was chosen. I began with the notion of forward momentum and that a ratio of four forward gears to one reverse meant that, to me anyway, it was designed to achieve forward motion. Once I began to identify the key components of the car it seemed that they almost made the connections to social work practice for me. For example the driver's seat could represent no other than the practitioner and the personal values that I bring to my practice. I had decided to utilise the wheels as the representation of the Aotearoa New Zealand Association of Social Workers (ANZASW) and Social Worker Registration Board (SWRB) membership which I connected to a sense of grounding and motion. This then left me struggling to come up with a suitable connection for the shell. I decided to read some more on the shell of the Mini and found that it was a unique monocoque design, which had made the mini so unique and iconic in comparison to other cars. It was reading this that I suddenly made a connection to Anti-oppressive practice. The uniqueness of the Mini's shell and the way in which it functioned made for a real easy connection with this approach. It was therefore the Mini itself that introduced Anti-oppressive practice into my practice framework! The connecting of components from the mini to social work practice became quite a lot of fun and I believe that due to the connection I had to the Mini it made the whole task a lot easier.

My ▫ Mini▫ Framework for Practice

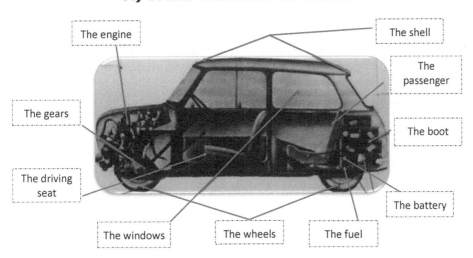

The engine
The shell
The passenger
The gears
The boot
The driving seat
The battery
The windows
The wheels
The fuel

Liam explains in the following narrative more about his choice of the mini as a metaphor:

The Mini was manufactured to be affordable for everyone from factory workers to pop stars. It was a vehicle that embodied equality for all, through its low purchase price, and as a symbol of change that captured the political and cultural climate of the 1960s ("The Mini", 2011, para. 1). Throughout its production, the humble Mini empowered generations of youth to be able to afford a first car that was economical to run and relatively simple to repair. I have selected different components of the Mini to symbolise elements of social work which I believe are important to the identity and uniqueness of the profession. These components are: the engine, which symbolises the theories, models and perspectives; the gears, symbolising the skills needed to engage with a client; the driving seat, symbolising the practitioner; the windows, representing transparency and personal reflection; the battery, the supervision; the fuel, symbolising journal reading and research; the boot, symbolising the importance of knowledge retrieved through client interactions; the passenger seats, representing the importance of good team/colleague interactions; the wheels, the Aotearoa New Zealand Association of Social Workers [ANZASW] Code of Ethics and the Social Workers Registration Board [SWRB] Code of Conduct; and, the shell representing a commitment to anti-oppressive practice (Cunnah, 2012).

In the exposition above Liam went on to explain in much more detail the rationale for his selection of components and their relevance for practice.

So what is a Practice Framework?

A Practice Framework is a conceptual map that brings together in an accessible design (Connolly, 2007, p. 825), the practitioners approach to their work. A practitioner practice framework is likely to include a combination of knowledge, skills, and values (Clark & Wilson, 2006). Students appreciate supervisors who are confident in articulating the theory behind the work they do in an unambiguous fashion, and are able to engage in discussions that link material covered in the classroom setting with how the supervisor conducts practice in the field (Testa, 2011). To this end, it is very helpful if supervisors have developed their own practice framework to use with students for supplementing discussions in supervision.

Cathie does just that with her Kete. . .

It (the practice framework) is useful to me but also to colleagues and students. I have it where clients can see it and ask about it and some do. So explaining the framework to them, refreshes it for me.

There are several compelling reasons for students to undertake the task of developing a practice framework as part of the placement supervisory process. The first and most important of these is to assist the student in interpreting the meaning and integration between their own values and beliefs, different types of knowledge used, with the ethics, policy and micro skills that inform their practice. Developing the framework facilitates a comprehensive understanding of the diverse components that contribute to social work as an activity. Secondly, having a practice framework enables students to transparently articulate what they do to others, including peers, potential future employers and educators, while opening up their own understanding of social work for both self-evaluation and increased public scrutiny (SCIE, 2014). This process models practitioner accountability. During the construction of his framework Liam starts to understand the notion of "use of self" in practice, and how this is integral to becoming an authentic practitioner. . .

It was through the development of my framework that I was finally able to see that, aside from the theories and models of others, the experiences, beliefs and interests that I held had an integral part to play within practice.

Thirdly, upon completing and presenting the framework to others students frequently develop a sense of confidence and competence about who they are and what they stand for as practitioners, contributing to an enhanced sense of professional identity. Finally, having examples of practice frameworks available for discussion in team meetings, online or during supervision encourages practitioners to consider their own approaches to the work they do, engendering critical discussions that contribute to ongoing opportunities for professional development. Cathie captures the evolving nature of changing practice and how this is reflected in her framework. . .

I keep it on my wall and it evolves now and then. The first version was a cardboard, printed version that I stuck things in. This version is a little more complicated. I'm toying with the idea of actually having a woven kete (using either harakeke [flax] or paper) that has the words on it so they are more fully a part of the kete.

The student supervisor, in their roles of educator and practice mentor is ideally placed to guide the process of helping the student develop a framework during the practicum. In order to overtly signal this task will be part of the student supervision, it is helpful to include the development of the practice framework as part of the initial placement learning agreement. Similarly, by having their own framework mapped out to show the student, the supervisor is modelling the importance of being clear about the factors that influence their own practice and how to use a framework. Having this discussion early on in the supervision process demonstrates the supervisor's ability to articulate the values and beliefs, policies and theories that shape the work being done in the placement agency. Developing a practice framework is a creative activity and as such requires time and space for the integration of existing knowledge with new ideas to occur. The extended duration of most social work placements, punctuated by formal and informal supervision make this activity well suited to complete during the practicum.

Constructivist principles are applied when using metaphor to develop the practice framework. Creating a metaphor incorporates an active cognitive strategy to integrate student practice experiences, knowledge and beliefs with a personal analogy (McAuliffe & Eriksen, 2011 cited in Deaver & Shiflett, 2011, p. 262). The process of generating the metaphor image involves cognitive synthesising on the part of the student, invites self reflection, as well as providing the means for others to explore the ideas within the image and provide critique.

A constructivist approach to learning entails students creating their own meaning and knowledge base through ongoing conversations, engagement with activities on a personal and social basis, and through use of critical reflection and interpretation of these experiences (Maidment, 2005; Giridharan, 2012). Comparing their own experiences, assumptions and understandings of these with others is part of the learning process (Andresen, Boud & Cohen, 2000) with the development of the framework as a whole enabling students to become creators and authors of their own knowledge and professional identity.

Where to Start

To begin the exercise of developing a practice framework the supervisor first needs to scaffold this learning. The notion of scaffolding refers to the means of support provided to the student to achieve the learning task; in this case the development of a practice framework. The process of educational scaffolding is contingent to the task, diminishes over time and is aimed at transferring responsibility for the learning to the student (Van de Pol, Volman & Beishuizen, 2010 cited in Van de Pol & Elbers, 2013, p. 33). Educational scaffolding entails providing clear directions to the student, identifying ideas and suggesting relevant resources, giving feedback along the way and incrementally introducing more challenging aspects of the task. The process of developing a framework includes engaging with the student in in-depth reflection, critical reflection and critical thinking. These processes do not necessarily come easily to students (Davys & Beddoe, 2009) and need clear introduction and structured facilitation as part of supervision. Ultimately the finished product of the practice framework will be unique to, owned and authored by the student. Liam referred to this awareness of growing professional identity and understanding about unique contributions being made to social work by different practitioners.

> Through the development of my framework I learnt that practice is adaptive and ever changing. Through utilising the mini as my metaphor it helped to remind me that social work practice is unique to the practitioner and that the sense of practitioner identity is key to the successful implementation of social work.

Images, or in this case the development of the practice framework consists of three stages: "process, product and interpretation of the product or process" (Huss, 2012, p. 1441).

As part of supervision a good starting place in the process of developing the practice framework is to use a whiteboard (another visual tool) for the student to brainstorm what the components of a practice framework might be. Although brainstorming is most commonly used in group settings, research consistently indicates that when individuals brainstorm on their own they come up with both more ideas and ideas that are often of superior quality than when groups brainstorm together (Mindtools, 2014). This is because within a group setting people get distracted by the ideas of others, rather than generating their own, or engage in a process of comparing what ideas they might have suggested with those already on a whiteboard. Individual brainstorming eliminates the worry about the opinions of others and therefore generates greater creativity. Individual brainstorming is therefore useful to use within and between supervision sessions. During this first supervision session the role of the supervisor is to encourage the student to put everything down on the board and later cluster ideas under broad topics, such as but not limited to, theories, ethics, legislation, policy, administration, key influences. Pictures, phrases or single words can be jotted down to jump start initial thinking about the contents of the framework. Having a range of different colours of whiteboard marker pens available is helpful as the student may intuitively use different colours for clusters of ideas that resonate in different ways. Prior to beginning the brainstorm indicate the different coloured pens, and note that during the brainstorm ideas can be connected using lines or drawings. Be sure to note that as a supervisor you are not looking for an artistic or neat piece of work.

During the brainstorm supervisors can prompt idea generation by asking the student questions such as: What theories do you most like, and why? What influenced your choice of social work as a career? What values do you hold dear? How would you describe your philosophy on life and work? What are the practice tasks that you believe are central to the work you do? It is important that the prompt questions are posed at a pace for the student to have time to think about their ideas and write or draw them up on the whiteboard. Supervisors need to encourage the student to stand back from the whiteboard and look at what has been written up. Does anything extra need to be added? A different visual perspective on the ideas that have been generated can be gained by physically moving and standing away from the board.

Once the first brainstorm has occurred the next step is for the student and supervisor to have a discussion about the items listed in the brainstorm. This discussion needs to take place immediately after the brainstorm. During the discussion the student may wish to add or delete initial points or make connections between ideas on the whiteboard. At this early stage of the process the discussion would simply be around the first impressions of the components on the board. If there were any glaring omissions, the supervisor might, through reflective questioning, prompt student thinking about these (for example, "I am wondering where organisational policy, or social policy might fit in your framework?"). Clustering of the ideas could begin at this stage under some broad headings such as ideology, theory, knowledge base, practice skills, values and ethics. In this way the initial brainstorm morphs into a mind mapping exercise. After this initial clustering the student then makes a copy of the brainstorm to take away.

Consolidating the Framework

Several weeks will be taken up with this next stage of the practice framework development. During this stage the supervisor guides the student to augment the initial ideas that emerged during the brainstorm. The scaffolding for this process includes suggesting readings to help the student refine the ideas; ensuring access to practice opportunities that will expand the student's experiences and thinking about what social work is about; providing the student with opportunities to network and engage with a variety of key stakeholders, such as colleagues from different disciplines, people from referring agencies, funders and consumer groups; prompting discussion in supervision that ensures the student engages in critical thinking and critical reflection about their work on placement and their practice framework; timetabling an event near the end of placement for the student to present their practice framework to others.

During this consolidation phase students are encouraged to use their practice opportunities on placement as well conversations with others to develop their framework. "Others" can include peers, family members, agency colleagues, individuals the student regards as significant in their lives for whatever reason. These conversations can occur live or online, with a few people or large numbers if the framework is posted on the internet for comment. These conversations do not need to end once the framework is completed as both Liam and Cathie attest. . .

> *I refer to it (the framework) a lot. I have shown my framework, in its text form, to all students that have been at my work place since I completed my studies.* Liam

> *All the time. I refer to it all the time.* Cathie

Principles of critical thinking and critical reflection need to be used as touchstones for these conversations, with supervision providing the forum for the student to test out ideas for the framework with reference to practice research, curriculum knowledge, personal understandings and professional experience gained on placement.

Generating discussions with "others" and the supervisor enables the collaborative production and interpretation of the framework. Components of the framework will be discussed and debated and finally conceptualised reflecting the pedagogical approach of constructivism discussed above. Repeated reflection with and without others enables student ideas to increase in complexity while facilitating the addition and integration of new information. As the student is working on what components to include in the framework, and entering into dialogue with others, these discussions will strengthen the interpretation of the framework and its links with the chosen metaphor.

The role of the supervisor throughout is on creating the links between disciplinary content facts and knowledge (in this case social work) and the development of new understandings by the student. This approach requires more than practice expertise and content knowledge of the social work curriculum. This approach to supervision and the development of the practice framework rests upon the supervisor being open to being creative and flexible in how the learning can occur; interested in the lived experiences of the student; having faith in the students own responsibility to drive their learning and to respect the student as a partner and collaborator in the learning process (Gilis, Clement, Laga, & Pauwel, 2008), as opposed to being an apprentice social worker on placement.

Formally Presenting the Practice Framework to Others

Presenting the practice framework in a formal setting to a team on placement or the class is an integral part of the student learning process. The presentation involves explaining the conceptualisation and interpretation of components, the metaphor and how together they illustrate the student's understanding and approach to social work. Furthermore, being adept, organised and confident in presenting to differing audiences is an essential skill for a social work practitioner (Regehr, Bogo, Donovan, Anstice &

Lim, 2012). As such the presentation in and of itself is a core competence to demonstrate as part of the placement.

Evidence provided by Vygotsky (1978) and others demonstrates that learning is a social activity. Presenting the framework, and responding to both expected and unexpected questions about its content and development, requires the student to draw on critical thinking skills in situ. These are skills practitioners must use every day to explain and sometimes defend their practice, advocate for resources and analyse issues of policy or ethics.

From past experience the presentation is a forum in which to both examine and celebrate the completion of the framework. It is an event that mirrors the dissemination of results at the end of a research project. If full engagement with this activity occurs, the student will have done a great deal of research to complete their practice framework. They will have learned how their selected theories, models, skills, policy determinants, ideology, interests, and principle ethics integrate. They will have learned about the application of this framework to practice. They will have learned how to be creative with generating an appropriate metaphor and linking this image with academic material. Most importantly they will have learned a great deal about themselves and how they want to be as a practitioner.

Conclusion

A key focus of student supervision is the promotion of a sense of student ownership, mastery and understanding of practice (Davys & Beddoe, 2009). Developing a practice framework can be a powerful and instructive method for promoting that sense of ownership and confidence in the practice milieu. Its creation and presentation to peers within the class and on placement involves a rite of passage, where the student transitions from "apprentice" to practitioner, in the knowledge that this is just the beginning of an exciting professional journey. As Cathie explained, the framework will change, as the practitioner experiences new and different ways to be a social worker. The quiet diligence of critically reflecting on ones day to day work and consciously adjusting the framework accordingly demonstrates an ongoing commitment to the profession and the clients it serves.

Acknowledgements

I would like to sincerely thank Liam Cunnah from Child Youth and Family, Timaru, and Cathie Withington from Presbyterian Support, Ashburton for their generous contributions to the writing of this chapter.

References

Andresen, L., Boud, D., & Cohen, R. (2000). Experienced-based learning. In G. Foley (Ed.), *Understanding adult education and training* (pp. 225–239) (2nd edition) Sydney: Allen & Unwin.

Clarke, I., Flaherty, T., & Yankey, M. (2006). Teaching the visual learner: The use of visual summaries in marketing education. *Journal of Marketing Education, 28*(3), 218–226.

Cleak, H., & Wilson, J. (2004). *Making the most of field placement*. South Bank: Thomson.

Coleman, K., Rourke, A., & Allen, B. (2012). Actively engaging visual learners online. *The International Journal of Technology, Knowledge and Society, 7*(5), 127–142.

Connolly, M. (2007). Practice frameworks: Conceptual maps to guide interventions in child welfare. *British Journal of Social Work, 37*(5), 825–837.

Cunnah, L. (2012) *Personal Practice Framework*. Unpublished assignment completed in partial fulfilment of requirements for the award of Bachelors of Social Work. Christchurch Polytechnic Institute of Technology.

Davys, A., & Beddoe, L. (2009). The reflective learning model: Supervision of social work students. *Social Work Education, 28*(8), 919–933.

Deaver, S., & McAuliffe, G. (2009). Reflective visual journaling during art therapy and counselling internships: A qualitative study. *Reflective Practice, 10*(5), 615–632.

Deaver, S., & Shiflett, C. (2011). Art-based supervision techniques. *The Clinical Supervisor, 30*(2), 257–276.

Duffy, T. (2005). White gloves and cracked vases: How metaphors help group workers construct new perspectives and responses. *Social Work with Groups, 28*(3/4), 247–257.

Edwards, S., & Cooper, N. (2010). Mind mapping as a teaching resource. *Clinical Teacher, 7*(4), 236–239.

Felder, R., & Soloman, B. (2004). *Learning styles and learning strategies*. http://www4.ncsu.edu/unity/lockers/users/f/felder/public/ILSdir/styles.htm. Accessed August 20th 2014.

Forte, J. (2009). Teaching human development: Current theoretical deficit and a theory-enriched 'Models, Metaphors and Maps' remedy. *Journal of Human Behaviour in the Social Environment, 19*(7), 932–954.

Gilis, A., Clement, M., Laga, L., & Pauwels, P. (2008). Establishing a competence profile for the role of student centred teachers in higher education in Belgium. *Research in Higher Education, 49*(6), 531–554.

Giridharan, B. (2012). Engendering constructivist learning in tertiary teaching. *US-China Education Review, 2*(8), 733–739.

Guiffrida, D., Jordan, R., Saiz, S., & Barnes, K. (2007). The use of metaphor in clinical supervision. *Journal of Counseling and Development, 85*(4), 393–366.

Higgins, J. (1994). Creating creativity. *Training and Development, 48*(11), 11–16.

Huss, E. (2012).What we see and what we say: Combining visual and verbal information within social work research. *British Journal of Social Work, 42*(8), 1440–1459.

Kadushin, A., & Harkness, D. (2002). *Supervision in social work* (4th ed.). New York: Columbia University Press.

Kolb, D. (1984). *Experiential Learning*. Engelwood Cliffs, NJ: Prentice-Hall.

Lakoff, G. (1993). The contemporary theory of metaphor. In A. Ortony (Ed.), *Metaphor and thought* (pp. 202–251) (2nd edition). Cambridge MA: Cambridge University Press.

Maidment, J. (2005). Teaching online: Debates and dilemmas. *Social Work Education, 24*(2), 185–195.

Marshall, J. (2007). Image as insight: Visual images in practice based research. *Studies in Art Education, 49*(1), 23–41.

Mayer, R., & Massa, L. (2003). Three facets of visual and verbal learners: Cognitive ability. Cognitive style and learning preference. *Journal of Educational Psychology, 95*(4), 833–846.

Mindtools.(2014). http://www.mindtools.com/brainstm.html. Accessed August 16th 2014.

Regehr, C., Bogo, M., Donovan, K., Anstice, S., & Lim, A. (2012). Identifying student competencies in macro practice: Articulating the practice wisdom of field instructors. *Journal of Social Work Education, 48*(2), 307–319.

Social Care Institute for Excellence (2014).The good practice framework: A full guide to the GPF http://www.scie.org.uk/goodpractice/files/gpf_full_guide.pdf accessed 18th August 2014.

Testa, D. (2011) School social work: A school-based field placement. *Aotearoa New Zealand Social Work, 23*(4), 14–25.

The Mini: a potted history. (2011). Retrieved November 3, 2011, from *The Telegraph* website: http://www.telegraph.co.uk/finance/jobs/4637660/The-Mini-a-potted-history.html

Van de Pol, J., & Elbers, E. (2013). Scaffolding student learning: A micro-analysis of teacher-student interaction. *Learning Culture and Social Interaction, 2*(1), 32–41.

Vygotsky, L. (1978). *Mind in Society: The development of higher psychological processes.* Cambridge, MA: Harvard University Press.

Walton, P. (2012). Beyond talk and text: An expressive visual arts method for social work education. *Social Work Education, 31*(6), 724–741.

Willox, A., Harper, S., Bridger, S., Orbach, A., & Sarapura, S. (2010). Co-creating metaphor in the classroom for deeper learning: Graduate student reflections. *International Journal of Teaching and Learning in Higher Education, 22*(1), 71–79.

Student Satisfaction with Models of Field Placement Supervision

Helen Cleak[a] & Debra Smith[b]

[a]School of Social Work and Social Policy, La Trobe University, Bundoora, Victoria, Australia;
[b]School of Sociology and Social Work, University of Tasmania, Launceston, Tasmania, Australia

Abstract

Field placements provide social work students with the opportunity to integrate their classroom learning with the knowledge and skills used in various human service programs. The supervision structure that has most commonly been used is the intensive one-to-one, clinical teaching model. However, this model is being challenged by significant changes in educational and industry sectors, which have led to an increased use of alternative fieldwork structures and supervision arrangements, including task supervision, group supervision, external supervision, and shared supervisory arrangements. This study focuses on identifying models of supervision and student satisfaction with their learning experiences and the supervision received on placement. The study analysed responses to a questionnaire administered to 263 undergraduate social work students enrolled in three different campuses in Australia after they had completed their first or final field placement. The study identified that just over half of the placements used the traditional one student to one social work supervisor model. A number of "emerging" models were also identified, where two or more social workers were involved in the professional supervision of the student. High levels of dissatisfaction were reported by those students who received external social work supervision. Results suggest that students are more satisfied across all aspects of the placement where there is a strong on-site social work presence.

Field education is considered central to social work training programs and substantial staff time and financial resources are invested to ensure that students are provided with quality field placements to adequately prepare them for the increasingly complex world of practice. Field placements provide students with the opportunity to integrate their classroom learning with knowledge and skills in a range of human service programs as well as offering specific models of practice for the future (Cleak & Wilson, 2007; Corey & Corey, 1997). It is estimated that students spend up to one third of their academic time in field placement (Fernandez, 1998) yet there is limited research available that examines the content of the teaching and the value of this practice learning for the student.

Field education in social work grew out of the apprenticeship model of teaching where students learnt by "doing" and the practitioner acted as a role model. This traditional model of field education is characterised by the placement of a student with a professionally qualified practitioner who assumes responsibility for professional practice learning (Cleak, Hawkins, & Hess, 2000). Much of a student's learning on placement is mediated through a student–supervisor relationship. This relationship helps to define and structure the range of student learning tasks and experiences. Contemporary studies of social work education suggest that the value of this practice learning continues to be recognised universally (Doel & Sharlow, 1996). However, Cooper (2007) challenged the old paradigm that field education can only occur in the one-to-one relationship between student and supervisor and suggested that learning experiences may be reliant on the core tasks and roles of the organisation where the student is expected to perform in a similar way to an employee. In a climate of significant industry and educational change, the one-to-one, clinical teaching model is being questioned as the most cost-effective method of delivering practice learning to students.

This paper is part of a larger research agenda on student learning in field education and reports on student satisfaction with key aspects of their field placement.

Background to Study

The field education components of most social work programs have become an increasingly complex and expensive process, influenced by two major contextual factors: industry changes, and education and training based issues.

Industry Changes
This study took place within the broader context of an ageing population, leading to a rapidly expanding demand for the provision of health and welfare services in community and ambulatory settings. At the same time, the Australian Government's agenda of social inclusion requires a vast range of services in the nongovernment, community sector to work with people who are excluded because of poverty, disability, or other life circumstances (Australian Services Union, 2007). As a result, training institutions have been under considerable pressure to produce greater numbers of well-educated, highly competent health and human service professionals to meet changing community demands, new services, and a forecasted workforce shortage (Australian Health Ministers Conference, 2004; Department of Human Services, 2004; Healy & Lonne, 2010).

Since the 1990s, the human services sector in Australia has had to contend with significant workplace changes, including the implementation of competition policy and the shift towards contracting services out, amalgamations, or downsizing of health and welfare services. Increasingly, management policies and political directions have embodied economic and marketing principles that have required health and welfare agencies to focus more closely on reimbursable and profitable services and intensified managerial control over professional labour (Maidment, 2003). Reports and surveys have highlighted massive turnover of welfare staff and the failure of the industry to attract and retain a skilled workforce (Australian Services Union, 2007). There has also been a significant change to the human service environment in Australia, with the movement of care of individuals and families into the community and an unparalleled prominence of regulatory governance to manage uncertainty and risk (Alford & O'Neill, 1994). These risks relate to the unforeseen issues of providing care and support to a range of people with complex needs, who now receive their services in a wide variety of settings in the community. The move to a new welfare reform agenda has also reduced government commitment to collective responsibility and shifted much greater risk to the individual, with professionals as key intermediaries (Ozanne & Bigby, 2007).

These changes in the human service environment have had a considerable impact on professional courses that are dependent upon them to provide field placements. A report published by the Victorian Department of Human Services (DHS) in 2008 identified expanding caseloads, an organisational culture and climate resistant to students, and the lack of physical infrastructure as factors contributing to the difficulty of finding suitable professional placements (DHS, 2008). Human service organisations that do not employ qualified social workers face increased levels of occupational stress and do not always have the resources and time to adequately support field learning (Beddoe, 1999; Hughes, 1998; Maidment, 2003). Bocage, Homonoff, and Riley (1995) reported a growth in work-based placements, a reliance on less experienced staff to supervise students, more requests for "good" students, and less tolerance for student difficulties.

A study of pattern and usage of field placements by all Victorian schools of social work between 1995 and 2000 showed a reduction in the number of placements offered by agencies that had suffered workplace changes, budget cuts, and had instigated case management targets (Cleak & Van Neuron, 2001). Difficulties in securing and retaining placements due to workplace demands and uncertainty in the field have resulted in a reluctance to undertake the added responsibility for student education (Cleak et al., 2000; Spencer & McDonald, 1998). The Victorian Department of Human Services has entered the debate and has commissioned a number of projects to identify the scope of the placement shortages in nursing and allied health placements and to begin to work with agencies and universities to try to develop strategies that address these issues (La Trobe University, 2006).

Education and Training Issues
Until the 1980s, most university courses in Australia had lower student enrolments, low staff–student ratios, and easier-to-teach "elite" students (Cooper, 2007). Higher education is now a global enterprise and Australian universities have been confronting aggressive government intervention through several cycles of reform for changes in teaching and learning quality, governance, student financing, and research (Ozanne & Bigby, 2007). This has resulted in mass education, declining

government per capita funding to universities, and escalating competition between institutions to attract and then resource these increased enrolments. In social work courses, the process of securing quality placements has become a complex and expensive process and is being made more problematic by increased enrolments and the large number of social work programs and other health and welfare training courses that require a field component. For example, in 2004, there were 1,838 social work students in Victoria, spread across six universities (DHS, 2004). Between 2000 and 2005, the number of placements required for La Trobe's third- and fourth-year social work students at Bundoora, increased by 60% (from 150 to 240), and the University of Tasmania reported an 85% increase in social work enrolments over the past eight years (Cleak, H., 2005).

Moreover, tertiary students now present with more diverse learning and personal needs, such as work and family commitments, access and equity issues, and language difficulties that require more flexible field placements experiences (Spencer & McDonald, 1998). As most students now pay for their education, they are becoming more knowledgeable about their contractual rights and the responsibility of universities to meet their individual and often complex learning needs (Cooper & Briggs, 2000; Maidment, 2003). Contemporary educational theories, such as adult learning principles and critical reflection, encourage students to be active participants in the learning process and to critically think about how their values and attitudes impact on their work (Gardner, 2006; Maidment & Egan, 2009). This context requires field educators to be skilled in using a range of teaching and learning strategies and to be open to exploring and critiquing their own practice. The Australian Association of Social Workers (AASW) professional educational standards also require social work programs to recruit field educators who possess the necessary skills and experience to develop quality teaching and learning environments for social work student placements (AASW, 2010).

These dual pressures from the industry and educational sectors have resulted in a struggle to meet the need for increased student placements in a "climate of resistance" from the field to undertake student placements. The recruiting and training of increasing numbers of field educators has also become a challenge. Some social work fieldwork programs have responded to placement shortages by pursuing academic-agency partnerships and the establishment of clinical schools in the health sector to promote collaborative teaching and research arrangements, as well as guaranteeing substantial numbers of clinical placements (Cleak et al., 2000; La Trobe University, 2009). A trend towards alternative work-based, interstate, or overseas placements has also been identified (Australian Institute of Primary Care, 2004; Bocage et al., 1995).

Changing Models of Supervision

Factors that affect students' placement experiences include the student–supervisor relationship, agency context, and the structure and nature of learning opportunities that students are exposed to (Parker, 2007). The quality of the supervisory relationship has been well documented as constituting a key influence on students' learning and level of satisfaction (Fernandez, 1998; Kadushin, 1992; Knight 2001; Marsh & Triseliotis, 1996). For example, Fernandez (1998)) found that students valued various components of the placement experience but the role of the field educator was pivotal to student satisfaction with their learning. Students appreciated structured time for supervision and capacity to examine skills, theory, values, and professional development. A study of 343 physiotherapy students undertaking their clinical placements in Australia were asked to report on their satisfaction with either group or individual supervision. Results showed that although most health settings use a model of group supervision, almost three times as many respondents indicated a preference for an individual supervisor because it provided more time for consistent supervision and assessment of the students and decreased stress levels for staff (Stiller, Lynch, Phillips, & Lambert, 2004).

Within the industry and educational context previously described, alternative field placement structures and supervision arrangements have gradually been introduced, including task supervision, group supervision, external supervision, and shared supervisory arrangements. An Australian study by Coulton and Krimmer (2005) showed that cosupervision, which is defined as two or more workers who supervise a student, is an efficient and beneficial supervision model and offered students increased accessibility to support and advice, greater breadth of knowledge, and diverse learning opportunities. Other models have been identified, such as the development of academic–agency partnerships and collaborative research arrangements, group, external, and collective supervision (Barton, Bell, & Bowles, 2005; Cleak et al., 2000; Cooper, 2007). Anecdotal evidence suggests that the use of external supervision by university or sessional staff is increasing and there is concern about the quality and viability of some of these emerging supervisory models (particularly external supervision) and whether they compromise optimal student learning. External supervision is a structure that is commonly used in field placements where there is no onsite social worker who meets AASW standards. Professional supervision is provided to the student for the duration of the placement by an external field educator, appointed by the university.

University field education programs have struggled to locate increasing numbers of quality social work field placements in a context where individual field educators are struggling to "fit" the requirements of student learning into their work loads. This makes it an opportune time to identify models that offer an alternative to the traditional, time-intensive, one-to-one model and promote optimal educational learning experiences for students. An analysis of 67 publications that discussed field education between 1980 and 1996 showed that the literature was dominated by research that considered the universities' or supervisors' perspectives but the experience of placement from the student's perspective was largely absent (Spencer & McDonald, 1998).

This study surveyed students' satisfaction with their field placements, focusing on supervision structures and models that promote or contribute towards positive learning outcomes. This particular paper is the first to report on the larger study. It examines a range of teaching and learning experiences offered in social work placements and reports on three aims:

1. To gauge the levels of social work student satisfaction with their placement learning experiences and opportunities.
2. To identify and document supervision models and structures used in social work student placements.
3. To identify models of supervision that promote positive learning outcomes.

A second paper will report on the teaching and learning strategies used by field educators.

Method

This observational, cross-sectional study was undertaken during 2006–2007. Data were collected from social work students, who provided retrospective ratings of their most recent field placement experiences. The study was approved by the human research ethics committees of the relevant universities.

Survey Questionnaire

A questionnaire comprising seven sections, containing both structured and open-ended questions, was developed to collect data. Each section concluded with a space for student comments, where students were invited to elaborate on their responses. A small number of final-year students (3) who had completed one placement were asked to pilot the questionnaire and provide feedback. Two slight modifications were made to the questionnaire based on this feedback.

Data for this report came from sections one, two, and seven of the questionnaire. Section one asked students to provide brief demographic information relating to their placements, such as the campus location, whether the placement was full- or part-time, and whether it was a first or second placement. In section two, students were asked to identify their placement supervision structure from four alternatives:

1. A social work supervisor who provided both social work supervision and task supervision;
2. A social work supervisor who provided social work supervision and a non social worker who provided task supervision;
3. A non social work task supervisor and an external social work supervisor provided by the university;
4. Other. Participants whose supervision structure did not fall under the other three models were asked to describe the arrangements made for their supervision.

This section of the questionnaire contained a preamble in which the terms "social work supervisor", "task supervisor", and "external social work supervisor" were defined. Section seven contained four statements that measured key aspects of the learning experience:

1. "Overall I was satisfied with the range of learning experiences and opportunities I received on placement" (Learning Experiences).
2. "Overall I was satisfied with the supervision and support I received on placement" (Supervision and Support).
3. "By the end of placement I understood the unique role of social work as a profession" (Unique Role).
4. "By the end of placement I began to feel some competence in practicing Social Work interventions" (Competence in Practice).

Participants were asked to mark the degree to which they agreed to the statements using a 4-point Likert scale (1 = *strongly disagree*, 4 = *strongly agree*).

Sampling Process and Data Collection

Social work students from the University of Tasmania and the Bundoora and Bendigo campuses of La Trobe University, who had completed at least one field placement, were invited to participate in this study. Questionnaires were distributed to cohorts of third- and final-year students during class attendance at the various university campuses, after the completion of their social work placements in 2006–2007. Students were given the choice to complete the questionnaires during class time or return them at a later date. All questionnaires were completed anonymously. A strong response rate (75%) was obtained from the 349 students who were enrolled in field education units in 2006–2007 at the three campuses. The retrospective nature of the study meant that while some participants answered the questionnaire immediately after the placement had finished, others answered the questionnaire up to one year after the placement had ended.

Data Analysis

Data were entered into SPSS (version 15, IBM, Armonk, NY, USA). Frequency data were generated for all items collecting categorical data (sections one and two) or ordinal data (section seven). There were small amounts of missing data for most items, in the range of 2–3%. Although the preamble to section two defined key terms, a very small number of students (2) misunderstood the different roles of the various field education staff involved in the placement and these responses were not included. Likert scale responses were dichotomised into *strongly agree/agree* and *disagree/ strongly disagree* due to the very low number of responses in a small number of cells. Chi-square analyses were then conducted to test the research questions. The significance level for the analyses was set at $p = 0.05$.

Results

Participant Profiles

A total of 263 social work students participated in this study and all had completed at least one social work placement, (both LaTrobe University and the University of Tasmania have two professional field placements.) Based on the responses to section one of the questionnaire, 77% of the participants were students of LaTrobe University and 23% were students of the University of Tasmania. Eighty-six percent of the students had completed their practicum on a full-time basis and 14% on a part-time basis. Seventy-five percent of the students reported on their first fieldwork practicum, 24% on their final practicum, and 1% reported on a repeat or third placement.

Aim 1: Overall Satisfaction with Placement Experiences

This section begins with a report on the student's overall satisfaction with key aspects of their placement. It then reports on relationships that were identified between campus location, placement type, and whether the students were full- or part-time, and satisfaction with key aspects of the learning experience.

Overall, results indicated high levels of satisfaction in the four key areas of placement experiences, with satisfaction scores of between 80% and 90% for three of the variables. The area where students expressed the highest level of dissatisfaction was in relation to supervision and support received on placement, where 26% of the students ($n = 68$) strongly disagreed with the statement.

Data in Table 2 suggest that student ratings of placement experiences were similar for the three campuses. This was confirmed by statistical analyses, which found no significant differences in the satisfaction scores on the four aspects of placement experience among students across the three campuses (chi-square analysis).

In relation to placement type, there were no differences in the placement experiences across first and second placement in relation to supervision, support and feeling competent in practicing social work interventions. However, students reporting on their second placement were more likely to understand the unique role of social work. ($\chi^2 = 3.9, df = 1, p = 0.049$). A significant trend was observed in the results, indicating that students were more satisfied with learning experiences offered by their second placement ($\chi^2 = 3.4, df = 1, p = 0.067$).

Students on full-time placements were more likely to understand the unique role of the social work profession than students in part-time placement ($\chi^2 = 4.9$, $df = 1$, $p = 0.026$). There were no differences in the other three ratings of placement experiences.

Aim 2: Placement Supervision Structure

Table 3 outlines the four models identified in the data. Seven responses that did not fit into any of the above categories have been omitted. These included three responses that identified different supervision structures across a number of placement settings, two responses did not provide sufficient information to clearly identify a supervision structure, and two responses identified a change of placement and supervision structure during the placement.

Table 1 Frequencies of Student Overall Ratings of Satisfaction in Key Learning Areas ($n = 263$)

Key Learning Areas	Learning Experiences ($n = 257$)		Supervision and Support ($n = 257$)		Unique Role ($n = 255$)		Competence in Practice ($n = 256$)	
	n	%	n	%	n	%	n	%
Strongly Agree/Agree	220	86	189	74	221	87	220	86
Strongly Disagree/ Disagree	37	14	68	26	34	13	36	14

Table 2 Relationship between Campus, Placement Type, Full-/Part-time and Satisfaction in Key Learning Areas ($n = 263$)

| | | Campus | | | | | | Placement | | | | Status | | | |
| | | Bundoora | | Tas Uni | | Bendigo | | First | | Second | | Full-time | | Part-time | |
		n	%	n	%	n	%	n	%	n	%	n	%	n	%
Learning Experiences ($n = 257$)	Strongly Agree/Agree	159	86	49	83	12	86	159	83	61	92	189	86	31	84
	Strongly Disagree/Disagree	25	14	10	17	2	14	32	17	5	8	31	14	6	16
Supervision and Support ($n = 257$)	Strongly Agree/Agree	134	73	45	76	10	71	141	74	48	73	163	74	26	70
	Strongly Disagree/Disagree	50	27	14	24	4	29	50	26	18	27	57	26	11	30
Unique Role ($n = 255$)	Strongly Agree/Agree	157	86	52	88	12	86	160	84	61	91	194	89	27	75
	Strongly Disagree/Disagree	25	14	7	12	2	14	29	16	5	9	25	11	9	25
Competence in Practice ($n = 256$)	Strongly Agree/Agree	157	86	49	83	14	100	160	84	60	91	191	87	29	81
	Strongly Disagree/Disagree	26	14	10	17	0	0	30	16	6	9	29	13	7	19

Model 1 emerged as the most common form of supervision structure. Approximately 55% of students used this type of supervision, which is most aligned with the traditional one-to-one student–social work supervisor model, consisting of one social work supervisor who provided both task and professional supervision to the student for the duration of the placement.

Approximately 22% of students received supervision using Model 2. Supervision was structured in a way that split day-to-day task supervision from "formal" social work supervision (i.e., one social worker provided professional social work supervision and day-to-day task supervision was provided by a non social work staff member).

Model 3 was identified from the data contained in the "other" category. A variety of structures were described by students (e.g., group supervision, split placements between programs, dual or shared supervision). Common to all was supervision provided by two or more social workers, who provided both task and professional supervision to the student. Approximately 10% of students received supervision using this model.

Model 4 consisted of day-to-day task supervision being provided by a non social work staff member and professional social work supervision was provided by a social work supervisor external to the agency. Social work supervision may have been provided by a social work staff member from the university or a social worker from another agency who had been contracted or had volunteered to supply social work supervision to the student for the duration of the practicum. Therefore, they were not staff members of the organisation or program in which the student was placed. Approximately 14% ($n = 35$) of placements did not have an onsite social work practitioner.

Aim 3: The Significance of the Supervision Model

The relationships between the supervision models and the key learning areas were assessed using chi square and a compelling picture emerged which is shown below.

Data displayed in Table 4 show those students in supervision models one, two, and three reported similar, high levels of satisfaction across all the ratings of placement experiences (75–96%). These models had both task and professional supervision provided by social workers only. Students in Model 4, where supervision was provided by an external social work supervisor, had lower levels of satisfaction than

Table 3 Models of Supervision Identified by Students ($n = 263$)

Placement Supervision Models	n	%
Model 1 One social work supervisor (providing task and social work supervision)	140	54.7
Model 2 One social work supervisor & non social work task supervisor	55	21.7
Model 3 Two or more social work supervisors (providing task and social work supervision)	26	9.9
Model 4 Non social work task supervisor & external social work supervisor	35	13.7

the other three models, with satisfaction ratings ranging from 49–71%. Results of the chi-square analyses were significant in respect to learning experiences ($\chi^2 = 9.3$, df $= 3$, p $= 0.025$), supervision and support ($\chi^2 = 14.7$, df $= 3$, p $= <0.002$), unique role ($\chi^2 = 22.4$, df $= 3$, p $= 0.001$) and competence in practice ($\chi^2 = 8.8$, df $= 3$, p $= 0.032$ respectively). In fact, less than half of students under this model of supervision (49%) said they were satisfied with the supervision and support they received during placement, compared with almost 80% in all the other models.

Discussion

There have been a number of significant findings of this study that are supported by the relatively large sample size, the strong response rate, and the collection of data from two institutions and three university campuses. Although the majority of participants identified a high level of satisfaction with their placement experiences, 26% identified dissatisfaction with the supervision and support they received during their placement. Results showed that students were more satisfied with their learning experiences and their understanding of social work than with their supervision experiences. In particular, final-year students reported a higher level of understanding of the unique role of social work, which could be linked to general preference by the field for final-year students as well as their interest and ability to work at a more autonomous and competent level. This study did not identify the actual aspects of supervision and support that the students were dissatisfied with and it would be useful to undertake follow-up study in this area.

This study identified three models of supervision that are widely used in field education. In addition, a fourth model, where one or more social work supervisors shared the education and supervision of the student, was identified from the student responses. Despite the context of increasing student numbers, increasing expectation of the learning environment, agency constraints, and increased workload demands, 55% of placements in this study used the traditional one student to one social work supervisor model. While this structure is labor intensive and places significant responsibility for learning and professional supervision with one social work practitioner, this model generally had a very high satisfaction rating. This may indicate the value that both field educators and students place on this model for professional learning. A follow-up study would be useful to explore and identify what it is about the models that students value and to more fully explore students' experiences of their learning on placement.

A significant finding of this study is the high level of satisfaction with Model 3, where two or more social workers are involved in the professional supervision of the student. This model uses a range of supervision strategies, such as group supervision, shared supervision, and split placement supervision, where students split their placements across two different agencies and had two different social work supervisors. These emerging structures may be a response to the effects of the constraints operating in agencies, with social work practitioners working together to

Table 4 Relationship Between Supervision Models and Rating of Satisfaction in Key Learning Areas ($n = 263$)

	Learning Experiences ($n = 250$)				Supervision and Support ($n = 250$)				Unique Role ($n = 248$)				Competence in Practice ($n = 249$)			
	Strongly Agree/Agree		Strongly Disagree/Disagree		Strongly Agree/Agree		Strongly Disagree/Disagree		Strongly Agree/Agree		Strongly Disagree/Disagree		Strongly Agree/Agree		Strongly Disagree/Disagree	
	n	%	n	%	n	%	n	%	n	%	n	%	n	%	n	%
Model 1: One Social Work Supervisor	121	89	15	11	109	80	27	20	123	92	11	8	122	90	13	10
Model 2: 1 Social Work Supervisor & Non Social Work Task Supervisor	46	87	7	13	40	75	13	25	45	85	8	15	44	83	9	17
Model 3: Two or More Social Work Supervisors	22	85	4	15	20	77	6	23	25	96	1	4	23	88	3	12
Model 4: Task Supervisor & External Social Work Supervisor	24	69	11	31	17	49	18	51	22	63	13	37	25	71	10	29

share the "burden" of student teaching and learning. This study substantiates the results of the supervision study undertaken by Coulton and Krimmer (2005), which confirmed the teaching and learning benefits of sharing the responsibility of supervision.

The other two models identified in this study had limited onsite social work input. Both Model 2 and Model 4 had a non social work task supervisor who provided day-to-day supervision and support to the student. However, there was a difference between the two models in the social work supervision arrangements. Model 2 had a social work supervisor onsite, whereas in Model 4 the social work supervision was provided by a social worker external to the placement agency. Model 2 had high satisfaction levels similar to those of Model 1 and Model 3; however, the level of dissatisfaction (across all key learning areas) was much higher for students in Model 4.

When these results are considered in relation to the different supervision models, it becomes clear that students are more satisfied across all aspects of their placements where there is a strong onsite social work presence. In particular, students receiving external supervision were significantly less likely to be satisfied with the learning experiences they received on placement, to understand the unique role of social work. and to feel some competence in practicing social work interventions. Although his confirms what students have reported anecdotally, the study did not investigate what the learning constraints could be. Drury Hudson (1997) categorised five main forms of knowledge that social workers use in their practice but found that they predominately used practice wisdom and procedural knowledge. External supervisors would rarely have the organisational and legislative background to adequately supervise students who are placed in organisations where the supervisor is not a member. Perhaps these findings indicate the importance of regular contact with and observation of student social workers practice on a day-to-day basis.

Conclusion

Social work is under pressure to respond to a variety of complex pressures from international and national higher education policies as well as demands from a changing human services sector. This study confirms the limited theoretical and emerging anecdotal evidence that a number of different models of supervision are currently being used as the field develops innovative ways to respond to these issues. The study also reinforces the superiority of field learning when at least one social work supervisor is present onsite. Further, it raises the question about the efficacy of using a model of teaching and learning where social work field educators are external to the placement setting.

Despite constraints identified in this paper, results suggest that the use of external supervision may not provide students with the most effective learning about the profession and practice of social work. While externally supervised placements appear "seductive" as they increase the placement pool, they are also costly for social work programs to resource and do not appear to be as highly valued by students as the other models identified in this study. Social work field education programs should be encouraged to resource the traditional one-to-one model of supervision as well as to explore alternative models of supervision that use collaborative arrangements between social work staff, such as shared placements, split placement, and group supervision. Further research to investigate the limited value of external supervision and the effectiveness of alternative models is warranted.

Acknowledgements

We would like to thank Dr Anthea Vreugdenhil from the University of Tasmania for her kind assistance with the data analysis.

References

Australian Association of Social Workers [AASW]. (2010). *Policy and procedures for establishing eligibility for membership of AASW.* Retrieved 14 March, 2010, from: http://www.aasw.asn.au/document/item/100.

Australian Health Ministers' Conference. (2004). *National health workforce strategic framework.* Sydney: Australian Government Press.

Australian Institute of Primary Care. (2004). *Clinical education review: Final report.* Bundoora: La Trobe University, Faculty of Health Sciences.

Australian Services Union. (2007). *Building social inclusion in Australia.* Carlton South: Australian Services Union.

Alford, J., & O'Neill, D. (1994). *The contract state: Public management and the Kennett Government.* Melbourne: Centre of Applied Social Research, Deakin University.

Barton, H., Bell, K., & Bowles, W. (2005). Help or hindrance?: Outcomes of social work student placements. *Australian Social Work, 58,* 301–312.

Beddoe, L. (1999). From preaching to teaching: Changes in field education in Aotearoa New Zealand. *Social Work Review, XI,* 21–27.

Bocage, M., Homonoff, E., & Riley. (1995). Measuring the impact of the fiscal crisis on human service agencies and social work training. *Social Work, 40,* 701–705.

Cleak, H. (2005). [Placement data, 2005, School of Social Work and Social Policy & School of Sociology and Social Work]. Unpublished raw data.

Cleak, H., Hawkins, L., & Hess, L. (2000). Innovative field options. In L. Cooper & L. Briggs (Eds.), *Fieldwork in the human services* (pp. 160–174). St Leonards: Allen & Unwin.

Cleak, H., & Van Neuron, D. (2001). *Researching the impact of the restructuring of the health and welfare sector on field placements in social work.* Conference paper presented at the Practical Experiences in Professional Education Conference, Adelaide, February 2001.

Cleak, H., & Wilson, J. (2007). *Making the most of field placement.* Melbourne: Cengage.

Cooper, L. (2007). Backing Australia's future: Teaching and learning in social work. *Australian Social Work, 60,* 94–106.

Cooper, L., & Briggs, L. (Eds.). (2000). *Fieldwork in the human services.* St Leonards: Allen & Unwin.

Corey, G., & Corey, M. (1997). *Groups: Process and practice.* Pacific Grove, CA: Brooks/Cole.

Coulton, P., & Krimmer, L. (2005). Co-supervision of social work students: A model for meeting the future needs of the profession. *Australian Social Work, 58,* 154–166.

Department of Human Services [DHS]. (2004). *Community health services: Creating a healthier Victoria.* Melbourne: Primary and Community Health Branch, Victorian Government.

Department of Human Services[DHS]. (2008). *Clinical placements in Victoria: Considering a clinical placement agency.* Melbourne: Workforce Branch, Victorian Government.

Doel, M., & Shardlow, S. (1996). *Social work in a changing world: An international perspective on practice learning.* Aldershot, England: Ashgate.

Drury Hudson, J. (1997). A model of professional knowledge for social work practice. *Australian Social Work, 50,* 35–44.

Fernandez, E. (1998). Student perceptions of satisfaction with practicum learning. *Social Work Education, 17,* 173–201.

Gardner, F. (2006). *Working with human service organisations: Creating connections for practice.* South Melbourne: Oxford University Press.

Healy, K., & Lonne, B. (2010). *The social work and human services workforce: Report from a national study of education, training and workforce needs.* Strawberry Hills, NSW: Australian Learning and Teaching Council.

Hughes, C. (1998). Practicum learning: Perils of the authentic workplace. *Higher Education Research & Development, 17,* 207–227.

Kadushin, A. (1992). *Supervision in social work.* New York, NY: Columbia University Press.

Knight, C. (2001). The process of field instruction: BSW and MSW students' views of effective field supervision. *Journal of Social Work Education, 37,* 357–379.

La Trobe University. (2006). *Clinical education reform options.* Bundoora: La Trobe University, Faculty of Health.

La Trobe University. (2009). *La Trobe Clinical School network: Outline of Model.* La Trobe University. August 2009.

Maidment, J. (2003). Problems experienced by students on field placement: Using research findings to inform curriculum design and content. *Australian Social Work, 56,* 50–60.

Maidment, J., & Egan, R. (Eds.). (2009). *Practice skills in social work and welfare.* Crows Nest, NSW: Allen & Unwin.

Marsh, P., & Triseliotis, J. (1996). *Ready to practice? Social workers and probation officers: Their training and first year in work.* Averbury: Aldershot.

Ozanne, E., & Bigby, C. (2007). Social work in higher education. *Australian Social Work, 60,* 1–4.

Parker, J. (2007). Developing effective practice learning for tomorrow's social workers. *Social Work Education, 26,* 763–779.

Spencer, A., & McDonald, C. (1998). Omissions and commissions: An analysis of professional field education literature. *Australian Social Work, 51,* 9–18.

Stiller, K., Lynch, E., Phillips, A., & Lambert, P. (2004). Clinical education of physiotherapy students in Australia: Perceptions of current models. *Australian Journal of Physiotherapy, 50,* 243–247.

Index

Note: Page numbers in **bold** type refer to figures
Page numbers in *italic* type refer to tables

127